PAGING Dr. Hart

DR. MELISSA DYMOND

The story, all names, characters, and incidents portrayed in this production are fictitious. No identification with actual persons (living or deceased), places, buildings, and products is intended or should be inferred.

Illustrated Book Cover by Qamber Designs

Photo Book Cover by The Book Brander

Character art by Qamber Designs and Hungrydamy (Etsy)

Formatting by KUHN Design Group | kuhndesigngroup.com

Copyediting by Dymond and Associates

TRIGGER WARNINGS

Death of a parent from cancer

Homicide/gun violence

Underage drinking in two scenes. The main character does not get drunk.

Teenagers committing crimes (theft)

Attempted assault

Please check trigger warnings. Your mental health is more important to me than book sales. XOXO, Melissa

Copyright © 2024 by Melissa Dymond, DO

All rights reserved. No part of this publication may be reproduced, distributed, or transmitted in any form or by any means, including photocopying, recording, or other electronic or mechanical methods, without the prior written permission of the author, except for the use of brief quotations in articles or book reviews and as permitted by U.S. copyright law. For permission requests, contact www.melissadymondauthor.com.

ISBN (eBook-spicy/open door) 979-8-9875850-6-1
ISBN (eBook-clean/closed door) 979-8-9875850-7-8
ISBN (Print-spicy/open door) 979-8-9875850-8-5
ISBN (Print-clean/closed door) 979-8-9875850-9-2
ISBN (Photo Cover-spicy/open door) 979-8-9903958-0-0
ISBN (Photo Cover-clean/closed door) 979-8-9903958-1-7

First edition 2024

Please visit the author's website at www.melissadymondauthor.com for character art, book deals, writing updates, and more.

CONNECT ON SOCIAL MEDIA—LET'S BE FRIENDS!

Instagram: https://www.instagram.com/melissadymondauthor

Facebook: https://www.facebook.com/melissadymondauthor

Tiktok: https://www.tiktok.com/@melissadymond6

Bookbub: https://www.bookbub.com/authors/melissa-dymond

*To every woman who's had her heart broken but still believes
in happily ever after, this one's for you.*

CHARACTER MUSIC

Tiffany: I Live in Patterns by Taylor Janzen

Ethan: Hey Girl by Stephen Sanchez

GLOSSARY

At the end of the novel is a glossary outlining the path to becoming a doctor in the United States. This includes definitions of the different stages of medical education.

DOCTOR

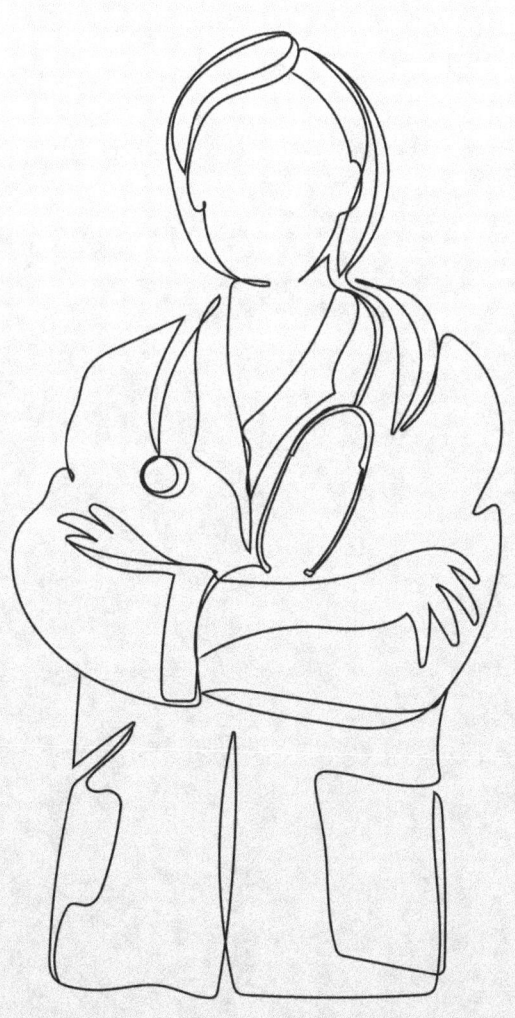

1

PRESENT, COLUMBUS, OHIO

Everyone's staring at me when I get the first mysterious text message. Because of course that's when it would happen. Not when I'm home alone or in my car or studying at the library.

Nope.

It has to be right then, when I'm about to start my presentation. The Mercy Hospital medical staff gathers in our auditorium every day at 8:00 a.m. for our morning educational conference. We take turns giving lectures about interesting cases, using them to teach the medical students and younger residents about disease processes and how to treat them.

Today it's my turn—my very first time. I'm not nervous, though. I mean, sure, my mouth is the Sahara Desert and my heart has crawled up into my throat, but I'm fine. *Totally fine.* At least that's what I tell myself as I gaze out into the sea of doctors. They look back with expressions that range from vague interest to frank boredom.

"Ladies and gentlemen," I begin. Heads swing my way, and conversation hushes. I've set my phone to silent. It sits on the podium, next to my laptop. I take a deep breath, about to continue my lecture, when the phone screen flashes and the phone vibrates so hard it skitters across the wooden surface. The noise startles me. I jolt and drop the microphone, which falls to the ground and lets out a squeal of feedback, like it's crying about its rough treatment.

Shoot.

Heat warms my cheeks. I let out a shaky, apologetic smile. The audience stares back, waiting for me to get on with the show. While I'm on my hands and knees, fetching the microphone, I wonder who the message could be from. Hardly anyone ever calls or texts me. The phone is still vibrating rhythmically when I stand. Acutely aware of the crowd, I peer at the tiny screen. The text is from an unfamiliar number, but the image is all-too-familiar. It's a photo of the iconic Las Vegas sign. The one you see when you first drive into town, right before you reach the southern end of the neon-lit Strip.

"Welcome to fabulous Las Vegas, Nevada," it proclaims in bold, blood-red letters.

That's…odd.

I grew up in Las Vegas, but everyone I knew there is long gone. I scroll down. There's no message, no name. Nothing to explain who sent the picture or why. A chill shivers through me, the icy fingers of the past walking down my spine. I inhale a shaky breath and glance around, searching the shadows of the room, but find them empty. Nothing lurking. Still, foreboding settles low in my stomach, weighing me down.

With the audience watching, I can't react, so I carefully school my features. I need to nail this lecture. Hopefully, if I do well, it'll win me the Resident of the Month award. I've wanted that certificate, with its shiny gold seal, since I first started working here three years ago. It's physical proof that I've transformed. More importantly, I need it for the $1,000 bonus that comes along with it. I'll give this same presentation at a medical conference in a couple of months. It's an honor to speak there, one not usually given to residents. The money will let me stay at the swanky hotel at Disney World, where the conference is being held, instead of a cheap motel 30 miles down the road.

Another glance at the text stirs dark memories, which I bury. With a sigh, I set the phone aside, refusing to think of it again. It's time to focus. Luckily, or rather unluckily, I'm good at compartmentalizing.

I've had *lots* of practice.

"A 56-year-old male presents to the emergency department with blood in his urine," I begin. Methodically clicking through my slides one-by-one, I outline how the patient was diagnosed with renal cancer. A CAT scan appears on the screen. With my pointer, I demonstrate how cancerous tendrils extend from the kidney and worm their way up into the biggest vein in the body, the inferior vena cava.

"For renal cancer," I explain, "we use tumor staging to help define the extent of disease and prognosis. Because the tumor extends outside the kidney, this patient is stage T3c." A click later shows photos from the surgery when the kidney was removed. Nearing the end of my talk, I discuss the patient's treatment and what imaging we will use for follow-up. This man will get repeat CAT scans every six months to make sure he remains cancer-free.

I pause to catch my breath, since I've been talking nonstop, and survey the audience. Everyone's still alert, and most are paying attention, which is all I can ask for. These early-morning presentations are often dry. Even I've had to fight to stay awake in this dark room when it was someone else up here lecturing.

"I'd like to open the floor to questions now," I say. There are a few raised hands from the crowd, asking about the man's long-term chance of reoccurrence and treatment options, which I answer easily. Relief floods through me. The finish line is in sight. There've been no technical difficulties. I haven't stuttered or said anything embarrassing. I give myself a mental pat on the back and prepare to end the presentation.

That's when a hand shoots up into the air.

It's a man, about my age, with ruffled brown hair, dark straight brows, and a square jaw. He sits next to Dr. Washburn, my residency director and boss. There's something mesmerizing about him. Something difficult to define but hard to look away from. It's partly his eyes, which are stunning, an unusually light color, warm amber like a glass of whiskey when the sunlight filters through it.

I've never seen him before.

I'd remember a face like that.

I nod politely. "You have a question?"

The man's voice is deep, carrying easily through the auditorium. "Yes. It's about the tumor staging. You said it was stage T3c?"

"That's correct." I frown, wondering where he's going with this.

"I think it's actually T3b. T3c is when the cancer is in the inferior vena cava but goes *above* the diaphragm. T3b is when it stays *below* the diaphragm. In those images you showed, the tumor was below."

Flustered, my normally orderly mind reels.

"Um—give me a minute." Time stretches out as I frantically search through the notebook where I wrote my research to prepare for this lecture.

Someone in the crowd coughs. Chairs squeak as people shift. The projector overhead whirs, its fan turning on. My breath comes in brief spurts. Hands shaking, I flip through the pages.

Where is it? Where is it?

Ah. It's there in my handwriting.

T3b.

The handsome stranger is right.

Darn it. There goes my award.

Heat rushes up my neck to splash across my cheeks. Humiliation gives way to fury. I'm mad at myself for making the error, but I'm also angry at *him*. Why would he correct me in front of everyone? Who even does that? I should have known. No man can be that pretty without also being cruel. Every eye is trained on me, waiting to see how I'll respond.

I swallow around the boulder in my throat. "It is T3b. I must have typed it wrong. I apologize."

"No problem," he says graciously.

Now, I hate him. First for pointing out my mistake and second for acting like it's not a big deal.

To me, it's a *very* big deal indeed.

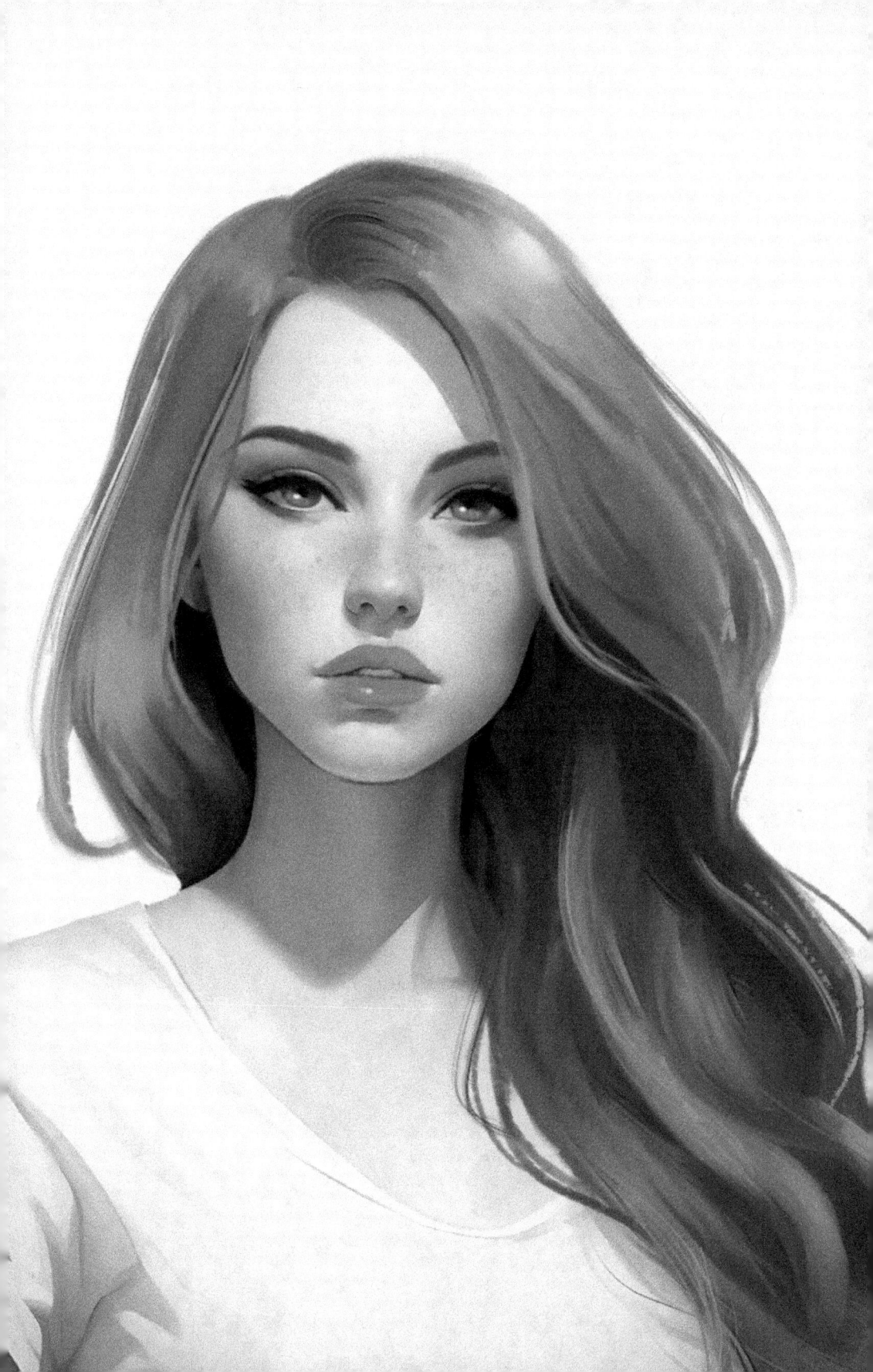

2

After the disaster of my lecture, I make a beeline for the coffee cart in the hospital lobby where I order my favorite drink, an extra-large, iced vanilla latte. Some people eat cookies or ice cream when they're stressed. Not me. My comfort binge is coffee. Once the cup is in my hands, I swallow a long sip, the ice cubes clinking against each other as they rearrange themselves. I close my eyes to savor the sweet, syrupy taste. A satisfied hum escapes my lips.

That's better.

"Hey, Tiffany, great job this morning," says a light feminine voice. It's Melanie, one of my fellow radiology residents. She has kind blue eyes, set in a pretty heart-shaped face. She gets in line at the coffee cart, with only one person in front of her.

"Yeah, right." Bitterness seeps into my voice. "I messed up the tumor staging."

"I didn't think it was so bad," Melanie says over her shoulder as she reaches the barista and gives her order—an iced vanilla latte, just like mine.

"Really?" I raise a skeptical brow.

Silver coins clink as she drops her change into the tip jar. "I doubt anyone even noticed." She gathers napkins and a straw before coming over to me.

"I don't know...." I trail off, doubtful. "Hey. Who was that guy, anyway?"

"What guy?" She smiles a wide, genuine grin at the barista when he hands her the drink and then shifts that same smile over to me.

"The one sitting next to Washburn." Together, we turn and walk out of the lobby.

"Oh, you mean the hot one?" Melanie takes a delicate sip.

"The annoying one," I correct, my eyebrows slashing downward. "Besides, don't you have a boyfriend?"

"I do have a boyfriend who I love." She places extra emphasis on that word. *Love.* "I also have eyeballs, and they noticed that dude is super good-looking."

I say "hmph" in a noncommittal tone, not wanting to agree but knowing she's right.

Melanie's pager goes off, saving me from the rest of the conversation. She glances down at it and then back up at me. "Gotta run. They need me over in MRI."

"Okay, see you later." I turn away, but Melanie's hand is on my arm, stopping me.

"Hey, don't worry about the lecture. You did fine. By lunch, no one's going to remember about the tumor staging." She squeezes gently. Usually, I don't like people touching me, but I tolerate her.

"Thanks. I appreciate it." I mean it. Even though we only spend time together in the hospital, she's the closest thing I have to a friend.

She waves good-bye, spins around, and heads in the opposite direction.

Drink in hand, I stride into my department. Going to medical school makes you a doctor, but internship and residency are the training that make you a specific kind of doctor. I'm learning to be a radiologist. As I walk to my office, I daydream about how wonderful my graduation day will be. When, after 10 long years, I'll finally be done with my medical education. Too bad that's still two years away.

The Radiology Department is in the center of the hospital, close to the main lobby. Its interior location means all the offices are windowless, a deliberate choice since radiologists stare at computers all day, reading X-rays, CATs, ultrasounds, MRIs, and other imaging studies. Sunlight coming in through windows creates too much glare on our screens.

When I burst into my tiny office, it's pitch black, just as I expect. What I don't expect is the deep masculine voice that rises out of the darkness. "Hello?"

Startled, I swear and jump back a step, thrusting my coffee out in front of me like a shield. I must squeeze the cup too tight because the lid flies off and the latte splashes over my hand, soaking my sleeve and the front of my white shirt. The sodden fabric clings to my skin, cold and sticky. I curse as I shake my dripping hand and aggressively flick on the light switch. The room floods with harsh fluorescent light, leaving the man before me blinking.

It's *him*.

The guy from my lecture this morning. The one who ruined it.

What the heck.

"You! What are you doing here?" I ask at the same time he says, "I couldn't find the light switch." Our voices clash into each other, warring for dominance.

A powerful combination of shock, fear, and anger has short-circuited my brain. I know I'm being irrational, but I point my finger at him. "What is wrong with you?" I demand. "First, you ruined my lecture and now my favorite shirt."

Stunned by my outburst, the man looks at me with wide, shocked eyes. "Sorry. I didn't think before speaking up at your conference. I noticed something was off with the tumor staging. Once I figured it out, I thought I should tell you."

His apology does nothing to cool my fire. "You could have kept quiet, but *no*, you had to point out my mistake before all those doctors."

"What? No. I wasn't trying to—"

Before he can finish, Dr. Washburn yells from his office across the hall. "Tiffany! My office, now, please."

"Just…hang on." I hold out my still-dripping coffee hand in the universal "stop" pose, like some deranged elementary school crossing guard. The stranger stands frozen, watching as I walk backward out of the room.

Dr. Washburn sits at his desk, dictating. He's a short man with ginger hair, receding and going gray. Silently fuming, I wait for him to finish looking over the X-ray in front of him. When he's done, I snap, "Who's that guy in my office?"

Dr. Washburn raises an eyebrow at my tone.

Quickly, I plaster a more pleasant expression on my face and rephrase. "Sorry. I mean, did you need me? You called for me?"

Dr. Washburn has a perpetually runny nose, either from allergies or the world's longest-lasting cold. Because of this, he always has a box of Kleenex on his desk. I grab a tissue and mop up my wet shirt.

"Yes, you'll be interviewing a candidate for our residency today. I sent him to your office. He's applying for the first-year radiology position. You know, Brandon's spot." There's disgust in his voice. Brandon had moved to do sports medicine in Kansas, and Dr. Washburn was still salty about it, not understanding why anyone would want to leave our residency. As far as he's concerned, radiology is the best specialty in medicine. "A doctor's doctor," he was fond of saying. "All the doctors in this hospital rely on *our* diagnoses," he would tell us radiology residents, puffing out his chest.

It takes a minute for his words to sink in.

Wait. Me? Interview that guy?

A headache has begun, a relentless throbbing behind my temples. I rub my forehead, hoping for some relief, as I desperately think of a way to get out of the situation. The last thing I want is to go back and face that man. Let some other resident do it.

Anyone but me.

"I have biopsy patients waiting for me. I don't have time. I—"

"Tell that first-year resident, Melanie, to do the biopsies this morning," he interrupts. "You interview the candidate and give him a tour of the hospital."

My mouth opens and then snaps closed. From experience, I know there's no point in arguing with Dr. Washburn when his mind's set. "Fine. Anything specific you want me to ask?" One more half-hearted pat to my stained shirt, and I toss the shredded tissue into the trash can.

"You'll figure it out," he says airily, flapping his hand at me in dismissal.

Back out in the hallway, I peer into my office. The stranger sits in my chair, swiveling idly from side to side as he scrolls through his phone. He doesn't see me. I turn on my heel and rush deeper into the department where the X-ray technicians and ultrasound machines are located, texting Melanie as I walk.

> *Tiffany: Hey, sorry. Washburn pulled me off biopsies. He wants you to do them. I have to interview that guy.*
>
> *Melanie: No worries. What guy? The hot one?*

Tiffany: The awful one.

Melanie: No way! Awkward.

Tiffany: Tell me about it.

Melanie: Good luck with that. I'll be right over.

Tiffany: Thanks.

Amy, the lead tech, is waiting anxiously, but before she can say a word I sail past, calling out, "Dr. Love will do biopsies this morning. Washburn reassigned me." Without waiting for her response, I duck into the supply closet and lock the door behind me. For some inexplicable reason, they always stock the small scrubs on the top shelf. I rise onto my toes and reach for a light blue set. Once I have them, I change quickly.

Melanie's already in the ultrasound room talking to a patient when I come back out. When she sees me looking through the window, she pokes her head out the door.

"Have fun with the hottie," she says, grinning.

I huff. "I didn't notice if he was good-looking or not."

"Sure, you didn't." Melanie sends me a saucy wink before slamming the door shut behind her. Even through the closed door, I can hear her laughter.

3

Back in my office, I find the stranger sitting in my chair with his long legs stretched out and crossed at the ankles. A ball of rubber bands, wound tightly together, usually sits on my desk. He's found it and is deftly throwing it into the air, where it rises slowly and then plummets back down, landing in his outstretched hand. He repeats the motion, over and over.

Distracted by the ball, he doesn't see me in the doorway. I take advantage and look him over. Brown hair with a slight wave. A tiny scar in his left eyebrow, a thin line where the hair doesn't grow. Faint stubble covers his cheeks, leading down to a cleft chin.

Life's unfair. He really *is* good-looking, in a boyishly handsome way.

I clear my throat as I walk into the room, causing him to straighten.

"You changed your clothing." He gives me a brief glance up and down.

"Yes, well, my shirt's soaked." I send him a pointed look full of blame. "So I put on scrubs."

"Sorry about that." His words tumble out. "I didn't mean to frighten you. Also, about your lecture, I—"

Raising my hand, I cut him off. "You know what? Just…forget about it." I sigh, remembering the dumpster fire of my lecture and that disturbing text message. "It's been a stressful day, that's all. In case you haven't noticed."

His shoulders drop, relieved. "I did notice. I also noticed that you swear like a sailor." A laugh rushes out of him, low and husky.

I blush and hate myself for it. "I didn't catch your name."

Seeming to recall his manners, the man stands, sending the office chair lazily spinning. He reaches out a large hand. "Ethan Clark. I'm applying for the radiology residency position that just opened up."

His handshake is like his smile, warm and confident. I pull my hand away quickly.

"Tiffany Hart. I'm a third-year resident." I feel silly about introducing myself. He saw my lecture. He knows who I am.

Ethan doesn't bat an eyelash, just says a smooth, "Nice to meet you." He flashes a brilliant smile, so handsome I almost forget to be mad at him.

Almost.

"Well...." I'm suddenly awkward, not sure what to do with this beast of a man in my small office. Ethan fills up the room, forcing me back against the door and making me tilt my head to meet his gaze. He's tall, well over six feet. It's all a bit overwhelming. I feel a need to remind him that this is *my* office. I'm the boss here.

"Why don't you sit, and I can start the interview?" I deliberately point to the smaller chair in the corner of the room. Ethan moves the chair closer and takes a seat. I almost feel guilty about how comically oversized he looks with his knees bunched up, like an adult sitting in a kindergarten classroom. I go to my chair, still warm from his lingering body heat.

"What do you like about radiology?" I begin.

"I like the challenge of it. How the images are like a mystery. All the clues are there . It's up to us to put them together so we can make a diagnosis. I like how fast-paced it is. You can help so many people in a single day. More than in a specialty like internal medicine." Again, that dazzling smile. I think he does it on purpose, knowing how disarming it is. Those white teeth would blind most women, but not me. I became immune to beautiful boys long ago.

Ethan leans back in his chair, seemingly at ease. "That's what I'm doing now, internal medicine, at Highview Hospital in Cleveland. I'm in my second year. Last spring, they named me chief resident."

I'm sure he's bragging about his accomplishment to impress me for the interview, but it has the opposite effect. *So arrogant.* I frown. "You're close to finishing your residency there. Why switch to radiology?"

That pretty smile of his fades. "I always wanted to do radiology. I originally applied to a couple of programs but didn't get in. Internal medicine was Plan B. Don't get me wrong, it's a great specialty. Just not for me."

This admission, that he didn't get into radiology on the first try, embarrasses him. I can tell. It's in the subtle ducking of his head and refusal to meet my eyes.

"How about you? What made you go into radiology?" His gaze travels over my face, touching lightly on my hair and ending at my eyes. There's a quiet curiosity in that look, an intensity that makes my skin prickle.

"Pretty much for the same reasons as you." I don't tell him about the hours I spent at my mom's bedside in the hospital. Or about the promise I made that I would become a doctor. How I swore to dedicate my life to healing others. Those details are mine, not to be shared.

"Will your current residency be upset if you leave? Do they know you're interviewing today?" Sometimes people do interviews like this in secret, not wanting to burn bridges with their current training program.

"My internal medicine director knows that I always wanted to get into radiology. He's friends with Dr. Washburn, so when he heard you had a position open unexpectedly, he recommended me for the spot." Ethan leans forward, closer to me. The room fills with a clean man smell, warm laundry and generic brand soap with a hint of mint. I inhale deeply, breathing in that scent.

His next words shock me. "It's going to be a resident exchange program. That's how it's going to work. I come here for residency, and the rest of you, including me, start doing rotations up in Cleveland. Two of us will go up there for a couple of weeks at a time. They don't have any residents in the Radiology Department at that hospital, so they need our help."

This is the first time I've heard of a plan to go to Cleveland, and I don't like it one bit. A particular little furry cat friend at home named Fred would object to my absence. He would be angrily peeing in my shoes for weeks if I left him alone for that long.

I scowl, annoyance rippling through me. "What I'm hearing is that *you* come here to Columbus and get your dream job. In return, the rest of *us* radiology residents drive three hours to a strange hospital to work as cheap labor in an understaffed department. Is that correct?"

Ethan stares back at me, not smiling anymore. Thunder clouds gather in that tiny room. Angry lightning flashes from his eyes to mine and back again.

He says, "I guess you could look at it that way, but that's not how I see it."

"Oh, yeah?" I arch an eyebrow in challenge. "And how, *exactly*, do you see it?"

"As the only way I get into the residency I've wanted since med school." He sets his jaw. "Listen, don't blame me. I'm just telling you what I know."

Like mirror images, we glare at each other.

It all becomes clear to me. This interview is a formality. If what Ethan says is true, then Dr. Washburn already plans to send us to Cleveland. Knowing him, he made some shady backroom deal with the hospital there. The mysterious text, my ruined lecture, my stained shirt, and now this Cleveland news. Can this day get any worse?

4

Turns out, it *can* get worse.

"Aren't you supposed to show me around?" No more smiles from Ethan, just a steely glare.

"Oh, of course," I say with exaggerated politeness, my tone saccharine. "How rude of me to forget. That's what I'm here for," I say, slitting my eyes at him, "to serve you."

I stand and go to the door where, overdramatically, I wave my hands with a flourish. "Please follow me." I flick my long, red hair over my shoulder and stomp out into the hallway without waiting for Ethan. But when I turn, he's there, right on my heels. Too close. He slams into my back with a muffled *oomph*. I lurch forward, windmilling my arms so I don't fall, and shoot an irate glance over my shoulder.

Rude.

"This is the Radiology Department. Down that hallway are the MRI and CAT scanners." I point to the left and right. "Ultrasound, X-ray, and mammography are down the other hallway. Nuclear medicine is downstairs." We make our way to the department's center. "This is where our administrators and lead technicians work."

The ultrasound rooms are empty. Melanie must be in between biopsies. I stop to introduce Ethan to Amy. He unleashes the smile on her. She stands staring, mouth agape. When Ethan turns away to peer into one of our fluoroscopy rooms, Amy catches my eye behind his back. "Wow," she mouths silently at me, motioning at him with her thumb.

I shrug my shoulders in response. He's decent-looking. So what? Doesn't mean he's a good doctor or even a good person.

Something about the way she's ogling him irritates me. I grab his wrist and drag him away. "Come on. More hospital to see." I haul Ethan along, leaning my full body weight forward to counter his large size. When he glances down at my hand, I let go, my hand and cheeks suddenly on fire.

We fly through the tour. It's easy showing him around. I've spent so many hours in this hospital I could do it in my sleep. Going up and down stairways, I take him to the Emergency Room, operating rooms, laboratory, and pharmacy.

By the time we're done, it's past 1:00 p.m. The growl of my stomach reminds me that all I had today was a few sips of iced latte before a certain *someone* made me spill the rest.

"You hungry? No tour is complete without a trip to the cafeteria."

"Starving." He rubs his stomach for emphasis.

The cafeteria is at the lowest level of the hospital. A slow stream of doctors, nurses, and technicians join us, all heading in. It's like watching a herd of animals migrate to the watering hole during an African safari. The greasy smell of char-grilled hamburgers and fried tater tots hangs heavy in the air as we enter. Underlying it is the chemical scent of medical-grade disinfectant.

I pick up a chipped plastic tray from the stack near the door. Ethan follows my lead, taking his own tray, and waits patiently behind me. We proceed down the line, grabbing plates of pre-made food as we go. When Ethan stops by the grill to order a burger and fries, I gape at him. "More food?" He's already loaded his tray with salad, two cups of strawberry Jello, and a turkey sandwich. "Are you really going to eat all that?"

A sardonic smirk from him. "Oh yeah. I'll eat. *Every. Last. Bite.*" He stares into my eyes as he draws out those last three words, letting silence build between each one. Something about how he says it sounds intimate, almost sexy. There's a weird hollowing in my stomach, a clenching low in my belly that has nothing to do with hunger. At least, not *that* kind of hunger.

"Besides, don't we get the food for free?" He breaks his gaze from mine to pile silverware onto his plate. "That's how we do it in Cleveland."

So entitled is the first thought that pops into my mind. "It's free, but that doesn't mean we should waste it." I wonder if this man has ever been hungry. If he knew what it was like to worry about making food last, stretching it out until the next paycheck came in.

A memory comes to me of my mother hunched over a pile of bills at our tiny kitchen table at night, a vase of wilting red roses next to her. Her calculator in hand and a line of worry dividing her forehead. How the spill of light and shadow from the cheap chandelier overhead turned that line into a chasm.

5

Once we have all our food, I swipe my badge through the scanner to check out. "Where do you want to sit?" I ask as we wind our way through the cafeteria, dodging tables and chairs.

"Anywhere," he says, holding his tray out in front of him. "Where do you usually sit?"

"In my office." I scan ahead. Half the tables are empty.

My comment earns an odd look from Ethan, his eyebrows scrunching together. "You eat by yourself?" he clarifies, like he can't imagine it. The idea of voluntarily eating alone.

"Yeah." My shoulders stiffen defensively.

We find a table in the corner of the room and settle in, sitting across from each other. Ethan bends over his plate, spooning Jello into his mouth. In between bites, he asks, "What's your story? Tell me about yourself."

"Not much to tell. I'm from Las Vegas, and now I live here." I don't dwell on what a relief it had been to leave Vegas. Falling silent, I start in on my food, hoping that will be the end of small talk.

I should have known better.

"Vegas, huh?" Ethan straightens, gazing at me with a spark of interest. "I've only been once, for a friend's birthday, but we had a blast."

I wince. "Let me guess," I say dryly. "You gambled and went to clubs." I've seen firsthand what kind of "fun" guys can find on the Strip.

"Yep." Ethan smirks. "Also, saw a couple of shows, the good ones with the acrobatics." A forkful of salad goes into his mouth. He chews slowly. "Do you go back there often? Vegas?"

"No." I give a small shake of my head, hating what comes next. No matter how many times I say it, this part never gets easier. "My mom passed away. I don't have anyone else."

You and me, Kitten. Us against the world.

"I'm sorry." Ethan frowns with sympathy. "I can't imagine how hard that must have been."

I nod, lips in a thin line, and look away, blinking rapidly.

After a heavy pause, he asks, "No one left there? Not even friends?"

Friends.

The word conjures an image of Shelly, not the teenage version with the too-thick eyeliner and dark lipstick, but the girl from when we were little. Those round cheeks and dirty blonde hair that turned to gold every summer, sun-bleached from the pool.

"No friends." Clenching my plastic fork so hard the edges dig into my fingertips, I fall quiet, finding comfort in the silence, wrapping it around me like a shroud.

Ethan fidgets for a minute, scraping his food around on his plate but not lifting the fork to his mouth. Finally, he exhales audibly. "Do you like radiology?"

I can't help it. A laugh sputters out of me. "Wow. You really are bad at this, aren't you?"

"Bad at what?" His straight eyebrows angle downward, half-offended and half-perplexed.

"Bad at not talking. Bad at sitting quietly." I take a sip of water. My almost-empty glass leaves a wet ring on the table.

"Maybe," he admits, somewhat sheepishly. "I used to get into trouble for it at school, talking to my classmates. By the end of the year, the teacher would have me in my own desk, off in the corner of the room, separated from everyone else."

"Did it work?" A corner of my mouth lifts involuntarily.

"Nah. I'd still yell over to my friends." He smiles at the memory. "It probably made me louder, not quieter. I just like it. Talking to people, getting to know them."

He turns his attention back to his plate, systematically eating his food like it's five-star dining. Which is crazy. I mean, it's hospital cafeteria food. We all know it's not good. Ethan sucks a dollop of ketchup off his thumb. My gaze snags on that motion, and, for some reason, my cheeks heat. To distract myself, I ask, "How about you? Where're you from?"

Almost all his food is gone. Only a couple of fries remain. He pops them into his mouth one by one before answering. He has a nice mouth, full and sensual. "I've always lived in Cleveland. My family's been there for generations. Both of my parents are doctors. The hospital where I'm doing my internal medicine residency—my dad used to work there."

I blink, unable to imagine it. That kind of permanence. Having all that family history to help tell you who you are. I had to make up who I am. It must be so easy for him. To walk in footprints his parents laid out in front of him.

Done with my food, I neatly arrange my used silverware in the middle of my plate and push it to the side. Ethan's finished, too. His plate is a messy pile of crumbs and smeared ketchup. He pulls a pack of peppermint gum out of his pocket and offers me a stick. I shake my head no.

This time, the silence is less awkward. He doesn't let it last long. "Listen, I know you're mad at me—"

"I'm not," I interrupt, straightening.

"Yes, you are. I don't blame you." His gaze is steady. "You're angry at me for interrupting your lecture and for messing up your shirt. You haven't bothered to hide your feelings, and I like that. I appreciate people who say what they think, who are direct."

Flustered by the compliment, I open and close my mouth several times, searching for a response. He holds up a hand, halting me. "I'm sorry for how we met, but don't worry. You'll get over it." He sends me *that* smile, the infuriatingly charming one, before adding, "I'm insanely likable."

My mouth drops open in shock. I retort, "Insanely cocky is more like it."

His smirk widens, unshaken by my words. "Not cocky." His eyes graze over my face in a way that sends a tremor through my body, like I'm having my own mini-earthquake. "Confident," he continues, lazily draping his arm across the back of the chair next to him. "There's a difference."

"Overly confident," I fire back, crossing my arms over my chest.

Now he moves forward, bracing his elbows on the table, eyes twinkling. "I promise," he says. That smile again, this time unfurling slowly. "I'll grow on you."

"Yeah." I snort and roll my eyes. "Like a rash."

He throws his head back, laughing like a little kid, so loud the whole cafeteria turns to us and I slink down in my seat, embarrassed. Ethan looks at me like I'm incredibly amusing, which I most definitely am *not*.

"Besides, most people don't like it." I stare at the floor, littered with crumbs, then drift my gaze back up to him. "When I'm direct."

"Well, then." He leans closer, his eyes sharpening with a strange intensity, and says softly, "Good thing I'm not most people."

We stare at each other for a moment too long.

Ethan's expression turns serious. He clasps his hands together on the table. "Be honest. Are you going to stop me?"

"Stop you from what?"

He doesn't hesitate. "From getting into this residency. You don't want to go to Cleveland."

I pause, secretly impressed by his boldness. Then I laugh loudly at the thought that I have any power in this situation. More likely, Dr. Washburn arranged this tour to waste time. To give Ethan's interview a thin veneer of legitimacy. "The fact that you're even here makes me ninety percent sure you've already got the spot. My opinion will have nothing to do with it."

He frowns, those expressive eyebrows inching downward. "That leaves ten percent of uncertainty. Ten percent that can change my life."

Oh, I get it then. How much this means to him. Back when I was trying to get into radiology, I was scared too. Worried that if I didn't make it into this residency, I'd have to choose a different specialty. I couldn't imagine it. Going to work for the rest of my life doing something that was my second choice.

I meet his eyes. "I won't block you. If they ask me, I won't sabotage you."

He must have been holding his breath, because now he blows it all out at once. "Thanks," he says softly, nodding in acknowledgment.

Before I can respond, we're interrupted by Melanie. Patrick, another first-year resident, follows closely behind her. They slide their trays onto our table and sit. Melanie darts her eyes to Ethan, then sends me a secretive smirk. I kick her lightly under the table, but she moves her leg out of my reach and grins wider.

The new arrivals pick up their forks and dig in. As much as I like Melanie, I have an equal dislike for pompous, boring Patrick. I make introductions, and Melanie strikes up an animated conversation with Ethan. She mostly covers information I already know—where Ethan is from, why he likes radiology, and so on.

Occasionally, Patrick interjects comments about himself. He tells Ethan all about why he chose radiology and how it is one of the higher-paid specialties. Apparently, no one ever taught Patrick that talking about money is impolite.

Now that I don't have to entertain Ethan, my mind returns to the strange text message from this morning. Who sent it and why? My mouth goes dry thinking about it. Hoping a drink will help, I get up to refill my glass. When I return, the atmosphere is strained. Ethan frowns down at the table with his jaw clenched. Melanie's normally jovial face is pale.

"Hey guys, what's going on?" I ask lightly.

"Nothing." Melanie's a terrible liar.

Maybe I should force them to explain what's happening, but one look at all those tense faces makes me pause.

For now, I let it be.

6

A few days later, during a break between patients, I'm looking at that photo again, the Las Vegas sign. It's been haunting me; a riddle I can't solve.

Needing a distraction, I decide to follow up on that strange lunch incident.

My fingers fly over my cell phone as I text Melanie.

> *Tiffany: Question. Last week? When new guy was at lunch? I went away and when I came back, everyone was upset. What happened?*
>
> *Melanie: Nothing.*
>
> *Tiffany: Tell me.*
>
> *Melanie: Don't worry about it.*
>
> *Tiffany: MELANIE!!*
>
> *Melanie: OK. OK. Don't yell at me. It was Patrick.*
>
> *Tiffany: UGH! He's the worst.*
>
> *Melanie: The worst!! Can't stand him.*
>
> *Tiffany: Same. So? What was it this time?*

Melanie: Talked badly about U. Told him to stop.

Tiffany: What did he say?

The cursor on the screen blinks its three little dots for a long time. The visual equivalent of Melanie hesitating. I imagine her typing out an answer, erasing it, and then typing it out again. Finally, the blue bubble pops up.

Melanie: Called U an ice queen.

Tiffany: That's all?

Melanie: Asked Ethan if he enjoyed spending time with the "ice queen." Sorry. He sucks.

Tiffany: It's OK. Other residents call me that, too.

Melanie: Not OK.

Tiffany: Been called worse.

Melanie: They're jealous. You keep acing our exams.

Tiffany: I study a lot.

The cursor flashes for a couple of seconds, and I wait patiently.

Melanie: Want to go out tonight? Some of us are going to dinner.

I sigh, already knowing my answer. Melanie won't like it, and I feel guilty about that. I wonder how long will she keep asking me to hang out before she tires of rejection and walks away. She wouldn't be the first person to give up on me.

Many times, I've almost said yes to her.
Yes to happy hour.
Yes to spa days.

Yes to becoming friends.

It's been so long since I had an actual friend. So long that I've been alone and lonely. I'm tempted, just for a moment, to accept her invitation. But then I remember how losing a friend hurts, how the pain echoes down through the silence of the days, months, and years that follow.

No thanks. Never again.

>*Tiffany: Appreciate the offer, but not my scene. More of a stay-home-and-read-with-my-cat kind of person.*

Again, the three dots form and reform for several seconds. I wait for Melanie's response. When it comes, I have the sense it's not what she originally wrote.

>*Melanie: Just don't turn into a crazy cat lady.*

>*Tiffany: I do have a cat…*

>*Melanie: Ha. Ha. Funny.*

I chuckle, picturing Melanie's expression right now. Bet she's rolling her eyes at me, with that trademark look of resigned exasperation.

>*Melanie: Sorry Patrick's a jerk.*

>*Tiffany: No biggie.*

>*Melanie: I like Ethan. He stood up for you, told Patrick he was wrong. You'd think he wouldn't want to ruffle any feathers since he was interviewing, but he called Patrick unprofessional. Said U deserved respect.*

>*Tiffany: Really??*

>*Melanie: Yep.*

I frown. What a strange thing for Ethan to do. We weren't really getting along. I certainly hadn't been very nice to him. Sure, I had agreed to not bad-mouth him to Dr. Washburn, but, besides that, I don't know why he would fight for me.

> *Tiffany: Weird.*
>
> *Melanie: He get the residency spot?*
>
> *Tiffany: Starts next week. Washburn just told me.*
>
> *Melanie: Good.*
>
> *Tiffany: Washburn says I have to train him, but I don't want to. Didn't really like Ethan.*
>
> *Melanie: Why?*
>
> *Tiffany: Too good looking and obviously knows it. He's entitled. He's arrogant. And he's way too quick to point out other people's mistakes.*
>
> *Tiffany: Also, not sure I'll be a good teacher.*
>
> *Melanie: Ethan's nice. You'll do fine. Need help?*
>
> *Tiffany: Cover biopsies again?*
>
> *Melanie: No problem.*
>
> *Tiffany: Thanks.*
>
> *Melanie: No worries. Remember, you'll be a great teacher.*
>
> *Tiffany: If you say so.*
>
> *Melanie: Hey, did U get Resident of the Month?*
>
> *Tiffany: Nope.*

7

PAST, LAS VEGAS, NEVADA, AGE 5

The small apartment I share with my mom is just minutes away from the famous Las Vegas Strip. The faint neon glow from the big casinos reflects on my bedroom wall at night. They're like a nightlight, comforting me when I wake up with nightmares, which is often. That brightness chases away the shadows in the darkened corners of my room.

It's been a magical time, just me and my mom. Days spent at the park or wandering the musty aisles of the local library. Nights cuddling on the couch with a bowl of popcorn between us, while she runs her fingers through my long red hair. Disney princesses promise happily ever after on the television. My mom dances with me around the kitchen, twirling us in circles until my head swims with dizziness, until my heart could burst from happiness.

Over the past few weeks, Mama has become more withdrawn. Worry etches the soft lines of her face, her eyes tight, and her words clipped. No more spinning around in the kitchen. Rose petals fall onto the kitchen table, and she doesn't clean them up.

"Mama's going to have to get a job soon, Kitten. Money's running out," Mama says.

This scares me. A job means I won't always be with Mama. I hate the thought of something stealing her away. I'm Mama's special girl, and we belong together, the two of us against the world. That's what she says, anyway.

She tells me brightly one morning, "You have a play date today. There's a little girl downstairs who can't wait to meet you."

I've seen the girl from far away and am curious. She always has a dirty Barbie doll clutched in her hand. I've been itching to get a closer look at it. As exciting as it might be to play with that doll, I still feel unease knot deep in my stomach. Mama spent the morning carefully putting on makeup. Covering her faint freckles with ivory concealer and twisting her blazing red hair into a spiral of curls.

"Don't touch! Too hot," she warned repeatedly, holding the curling iron far away.

I think my mother is beautiful, like one of those cartoon princesses. I'm not the only one who sees it. Strangers turn their heads to watch her walk through the grocery store. Men stare at her long, slim legs. Before today I thought my mama didn't care about her looks, maybe didn't even realize she was so pretty. Now I'm not sure. The easy way she applied her lipstick and fluffed up her hair made it seem like she's done it before, many times. There's something unrecognizable in this painted version of Mama. I don't trust it.

After slipping into some brand new clickity-clack heels, Mama takes my hand. We walk together down the stairs to knock on the neighbor's door, which opens to reveal a lady with hair dyed so blonde it's almost white. There's a faint line of darker roots at the base of her hair, contrasting against overly tan skin.

Mama bends down to my level. Her hazel-green eyes are the same shade as mine. "Baby, this here is Ms. Brandi. She's going to look after you today. You be a good girl for her and listen to what she says. Okay?"

I nod solemnly. She doesn't ask for much, so I'm eager to please. I gulp against the fear choking my throat. "Are you coming back soon?" I have a sudden terrifying thought that I may never see her again.

"Of course, Kitten. I won't be gone too long. Don't you worry." Mom looks away quickly but not before I see the faint sheen of unshed tears in her eyes. That makes me want to cry too, but I'm a big girl so I don't.

My mom stands to talk to Ms. Brandi, and now I see the little girl peering curiously around her mother's legs. She stares openly at me, brown eyes scanning me from head to toe. A warm smile breaks over her face as she steps out into the doorway with a quiet, "Hi."

"Hi." I'm suddenly shy. I've played with kids at the park before but never spent more than an hour or two with another child. I'm not sure what the rules of friendship are. Do we hug? Share each other's lunch? I try to think of the movies and TV shows I've watched for clues but come up blank.

Luckily, the other girl is more self-assured. She grabs my hand with sticky fingers and pulls me deeper into the apartment. "Come see my toys," she shouts over her shoulder as she drags me along. A thrill of excitement tingles through me. I'm bored with all my toys at home. The thought of playing with something new distracts me so much that I barely hear Mama call out good-bye before the door closes.

"I'm Shelly. What's your name?" asks the girl as we walk into her room.

"Tiffany," I answer, looking around in awe. It's pretty and girly in here, with pink-painted walls and a ruffled bedspread.

"I thought maybe your name was Kitten, because that's what your mom said." Shelly tilts her head, a tiny wrinkle forming between her brows.

For the first time, I'm embarrassed by my nickname. "No, that's just something my mama calls me."

"Oh. Too bad. That would be a cool name. Cats are my favorite animal. What's your favorite? Do you want to play kittens?" The little girl speaks lightning fast. I have to concentrate to follow her words.

"Sure. How do we play?" I look around for some cat stuffed animals or toys.

"We pretend, silly!" Shelly gets down on her hands and knees and makes surprisingly realistic meowing sounds.

A grin stretches over my face. My mom plays with me all the time but not games like this. I've always wanted a cat, but Mama says the apartment manager won't let us. I copy Shelly's movements, and soon we're roaming around the room, purring and pretending to lick our paws.

We spend hours playing together. Barbies, Hot Wheels, hide and seek. In the middle of the day, Brandi feeds us peanut butter and jelly sandwiches with bright orange Cheetos. It's my first-time eating the crunchy chips. I watch with fascination as Shelly sucks the thick cheese powder off her fingers one by one. Imitating her, I lick my fingers clean.

Brandi gives us popsicles for dessert. She lets us each pick our favorite color. Shelly takes red, and I choose purple. Brandi shoos us outside with the frozen treats, saying, "Don't you dare spill and make my floors sticky. Get out, you two."

I don't mention that Brandi's floors are already sticky. My mama taught me manners. My mama says, "If you can't say something nice, then don't say anything at all."

Outside, we sit shoulder to shoulder on the stained concrete steps that lead up to my apartment. Sighing happily, I tip the melted grape popsicle into my mouth.

"Where's your daddy?" asks Shelly out of the blue.

"I don't have one." Popsicle juice spills onto my hand, and I lick it off.

She laughs, an adult laugh. "Everyone has a daddy. Mine went away. Mommy says he's no good."

I've seen some dads around, but my mama has been with me so much that I never felt the need for one. I haven't stopped to consider where mine might be.

The sound of heels on concrete makes us look up. Mom's home. She looks tired but triumphant. I jump up, leaving the empty popsicle wrapper behind me on the ground, forgotten. I fly to Mama and hug her legs.

Suddenly I'm crying. I don't know why. I've been having fun with Shelly, but seeing Mama releases a weight I didn't know I was carrying. It crashes down around me. The thought of someday losing her reoccurs, and I sob jaggedly.

Brandi comes outside to see what the commotion is all about. "Goodness!" she exclaims when she sees my tear-streaked face. "I swear she was fine a minute ago," she tells Mom and shoots me an irritated glare.

Mama scoops me up into her arms and rocks me like I'm a toddler. I'm too upset to care that I'm being treated like a younger child instead of the big five-year-old girl that I am. I wrap my legs around Mama's waist and bury my face in her neck. She smells sweet, like wild roses.

Rubbing a comforting hand on my back, Mom tells Brandi, "I'm sure she's just tired. It's been a big day for her."

My mom talks to Brandi for a few more minutes and then carries me upstairs. We snuggle together on the old worn-out plaid couch for the rest of the night. I keep a close eye on her, following her into the bathroom and kitchen the few times she leaves the room.

Later, Mama tells me, "I got a job today, Kitten. I'm going to work in that big casino we drive past sometimes. You know, the fancy one with the marble columns in the front that looks like it's from Italy. Ms. Brandi will watch you in the daytime when I'm gone. Then I'm going to watch Shelly here at our place when Brandi works at night. Won't that be fun? You'll finally have someone to play with."

I don't know what to think about this. I like Shelly but hate to be away from Mama. "Do you have to?" I ask in a plaintive voice.

She sighs. "Yes, honey, I do."

As she tucks me into bed that night, I suddenly remember. "Mama, where's my daddy?"

She steps back, a glimmer of alarm passing over her so quickly I almost miss it. She's quiet for a moment, thinking. Finally, she says, "He died. It was a long time ago. I'm sorry, Kitten."

That night I cry in the dark for a father I'll never meet.

8

PAST, LAS VEGAS, NEVADA, AGE 8

Shelly and I grow up together like sisters. Days at Shelly's apartment and nights at mine. It's odd because our moms aren't good friends. They rarely spend time together when they're both off work. It's more like they're co-parents, disgruntled ex's who share the burden of child care, each slightly disapproving of the other's child-rearing methods.

Sometimes Mom whispers, "Brandi, if that's even her real name," under her breath. My mom frowns as she washes Oreo and Cheetos dust off my fingers at night. A gummy multivitamin makes its way onto Shelly's and my plates at dinner, along with our homemade fettucine Alfredo. Mama tries to school the wildness out of us, especially Shelly. She teaches us table manners and some fancy word I can't pronounce...etiquette. She shows us how to "walk like a lady," which involves prancing around the apartment with books balanced on our heads. I get up to three books before they topple to the floor.

For her part, Brandi is bothered by my mom's lack of a man. She brings it up one day in late spring, when the weather is already scorching hot. We're all at the apartment pool together. Mom slathers us both in sunscreen, ranting about how our fair skin needs extra protection and I will thank her for this later.

I squirm under my mother's slick hands, eager to join Shelly, who's already cannon balled into the pool. Once I get into the shallow end, Shelly and I take turns seeing how long we can hold our breath underwater. Shelly is 42 seconds, and I'm a proud 48 seconds. Shelly's mad I beat her. She complains I cheated and angrily splashes water in my face, which makes my eyes sting. Tears mix with water droplets that run down my cheeks.

The moms talk in hushed tones at the side of the pool, stretched out next to each other on chaise lounge chairs. The cheap kind, with thin plastic strips that dig into your back. I swim closer, eavesdropping as Brandi asks my mom if she'll start dating soon.

"I don't think so," replies Mama absently. She thumbs her way through the thick book in her hands. She's always reading novels, my mama. The other moms all read magazines with glossy covers and skinny women wearing bright red lipstick on the front. Sometimes, I wish she would try to blend in a little more. Pick up a magazine or highlight her hair. I'm starting to notice things like that. How my mother sticks out in this place, a red rose among a bunch of carnations.

Brandi unties her bikini top and lets it drop to the ground. I avert my eyes, to avoid looking at her giant beach ball–rounded breasts. I can't explain why, but seeing her naked chest makes me feel uncomfortable, like I'm doing something wrong, looking at something I shouldn't. All she wears now is a tiny string bikini bottom. She rubs tanning oil over her arms and chest, gleaming blindingly in the sun.

I've asked Mom before why Brandi and some of the other apartment ladies wear so little when they sit out sunbathing at the pool. After a long pause, she says, "They can't have tan lines for their job." My mother refused to explain any further.

Brandi shoots my mom an incredulous look and whispers, rather loudly, "But what about the sex? Don't you miss it?"

My mom's lips thin into a disapproving line. "Not at all."

Brandi's eyes pop open even wider, and she says with equal disapproval, "Then you obviously weren't doing it right."

TEACHER

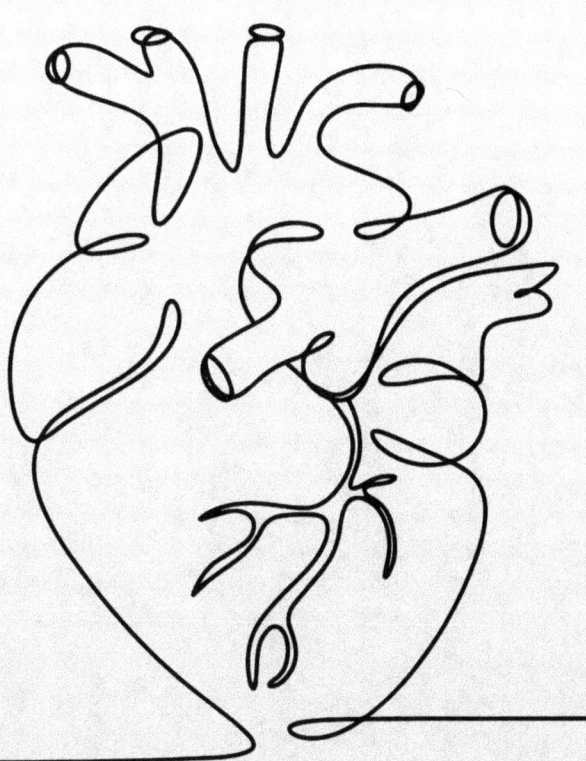

9

PRESENT, COLUMBUS, OHIO

The next week, I train Ethan. We're in the ultrasound department, where the rooms are so small that the bulky ultrasound machine and the patient in a rolling hospital bed barely fit. Whenever Ethan, the ultrasound technician, Jill, or I maneuver around the room, we call out our movements so we don't bump into one another.

"On your right. Watch your toes," says Jill, as she rolls her stool closer to the patient.

I have a plan for today. After giving it serious thought over the weekend, I've decided to take a different approach with Ethan. He defended me to Patrick so I might owe him, which is an uncomfortable thought. I make a mental promise to be extra kind to pay him back.

My "niceness plan" crashes into burning flames ten minutes later.

I'm teaching Ethan how to do an ultrasound-guided paracentesis, a procedure to treat ascites, a condition where abnormal fluid accumulates in a patient's belly, making it swell up like a balloon. To treat this, we use a long needle to insert a flexible tube into the patient's abdomen. The tube acts like a big straw and sucks out the extra fluid.

Ethan's being an ass and resisting my instructions.

"I already know how to do this," he grumbles, frustrated as I explain the procedure for the third time. "I was on a GI rotation for a month and did like a hundred of these."

He sounds like a whiny three-year-old. I want to smack him on the butt and not in a sexy kind of way. "I'm sure you did these before, but not with the ultrasound machine. The GI doctors do them blind." I count to ten slowly and continue. "In GI, they stick the tube in anywhere. Here in radiology, we use ultrasound to help us. It's better because we can see inside the patient. We can locate the biggest pocket of fluid to target. That way there's less chance of complications."

"We never had complications in GI when we did it without ultrasound," Ethan shoots back.

Thank goodness the patient is too out of it to hear us bicker. It can't be very confidence-inspiring to watch your doctors argue. It's already bad enough that Jill's in the room with us. Her eyes bounce back and forth like we're the best tennis match at Wimbledon. Gossip travels quicker than wildfire in the hospital, which means everyone will know that Ethan and I are proverbial oil and water.

"Well, you're not in GI anymore. You're in radiology, so act like a radiologist already!" I shove the ultrasound probe into his hand. I angrily grab that hand and place it on the patient's distended belly.

Gray and black images pop up on the ultrasound computer screen. To the untrained eye, it looks like a swirling snowstorm of monochromatic pixels. To me, it looks like the inside of the patient's body. I can clearly see his internal organs and the abnormal fluid.

The images shift as I guide his hand along the patient's skin. I'm pressed up against Ethan, who sits in a chair while I stand behind him, staring at the screen over his shoulder. When I talk, my breath stirs the hair on the nape of his neck. Goosebumps break out along his skin, and he shivers.

Is the air conditioning too strong?

Ethan's protests fade as he takes in the picture before him. He leans forward, staring at the screen with an expression of wonder.

"See those gray pulsing tubes? Those are the intestines. They're moving because of peristalsis, which helps the food pass through," I explain as I move his hand lower on the patient's abdomen. "Now look down here. At these big black spaces. That's the fluid. When the patient lies on their back, gravity pulls it down low."

"Wow. That's cool." Ethan's impressed, his eyes wide and jaw slack. "I've seen ultrasounds of the gallbladder and stuff like that before, but it was just static frozen images. Not in real-time like this. This is like the difference between looking at a photo versus watching a movie."

I relax, letting the joy of my work sweep me away. "I know. It's pretty neat, isn't it? It's like being Superman and having X-ray vision. We get to see right into the center of people." Lots of days medicine is a grueling job, but moments like this make all the sacrifice worth it. Ethan twists in his seat to look at me. We exchange wide grins with each other, both high on the miracle of modern medicine.

I point at the screen. "Right there. That's where we'll get the best result."

After we pick the spot, I instruct Ethan on how to cleanse and numb the patient's skin. With my hands over his again, I help him guide the needle through the abdominal wall and into the fluid. We attach the tube to a suction bottle. Immediately, clear yellow liquid pours in. When that bottle is full, we replace it with another. We continue this process until the patient's belly deflates like a punctured tire.

"Seven liters total removed," I say, proudly holding up the last fluid-filled bottle.

Ethan stares at it in awe. "It's crazy that someone can walk around with all that sloshing inside of them."

I nod in agreement, pulling off my glasses, the ones I use when I need to see something close up. "Mr. Adams is going to feel better when he wakes up and realizes this is all gone. He's going to breathe easier. That big belly pushes up on his chest, making it hard to take a deep breath."

After bandaging the tiny wound from the tube, we exit the patient's room. The incessant beeping of monitors surrounds us as we walk through the ICU.

"You were really great in there," Ethan says, his eyes shining.

"Well, I've had lots of practice. Being a doctor is basically my whole life." Usually, that thought makes me happy, but somehow speaking it out loud to Ethan makes it sound hollow. I realize with a start that if I lost this job I would have nothing. It's become my whole identity, the thing I wake up for in the morning.

My phone dings in my pocket as we exit the double doors of the ICU. When I look at what's on the screen, a shudder runs through me.

Ethan can't see this.

I angle the phone away from him, hiding the text. It's from that same person, the one I don't know. I had thought about blocking the number after the last disturbing message but decided against it. I hoped it had been a fluke, that Las Vegas picture. Maybe it was a random one-off, a coincidence. Apparently, I was in denial. Today's text is an image of a gambling chip, the kind you use to bet in a casino. The Statue of Liberty in its center and around its red edge, it reads $5 New York-New York Hotel and Casino, Las Vegas, NV.

My shock must be obvious because Ethan is asking, "Tiffany? Everything okay?" He places his hand lightly on my upper arm, the warmth of his touch burning through the sleeve of my lab coat.

"Oh, yes. Fine." I quickly adjust my expression, slipping my calm, professional mask on. I've slowed my walk while I looked at my phone. Now I speed forward, moving so fast that Ethan has to stretch out his long legs to keep up. We enter the elevator on our way down to the Radiology Department.

My mind whirs, obsessing over the text. What does it mean? Who could have sent it and why? There's a sinking sensation, a feeling of dread, as I consider the possibilities. I'm so lost in my thoughts that it takes a second to recognize Ethan's talking to me.

"About earlier, with the ultrasound patient…" He clears his throat and stabs at the first-floor button. The elevator jolts, making my stomach drop, and begins its descent. "I should have listened to you. It's just kind of hard," he mumbles, staring down at his feet. "I spent almost two years in internal medicine. I had enough experience that I knew what I was doing, the diagnoses and how to treat them. Now I'm back to square one. I'm glad to finally be in radiology, but it's frustrating to start all over again." His eyes slide up to mine, then skitter away. "Anyway, sorry."

His apology is the last thing I was expecting. I hadn't given much consideration to how it must feel, being the "new kid" again. Hate to admit it, but I'm impressed by his honesty. "It's okay. Nobody's perfect," I reassure him, wanting to ease his tension.

Somewhere in the shadowy hallways of my past, neon lights flicker, gunshots ring out, and glass shatters, reminding me exactly how *not* perfect I am. Ethan has no idea about the mistakes I've made.

No one does.

10

PAST, LAS VEGAS, NEVADA, AGE 10

In the summer, a guy named Mike starts to hang around Brandi's place. He's younger than Brandi. Good-looking in an unkempt way. String-bean thin with a lightly muscled body that he likes to show off with tight, heavy metal-band t-shirts. During the day, Mike works on cars. At night, he works security at the club where Brandi works.

Brandi is the happiest I have ever seen. She walks around singing and shaking her full hips from side to side. Surprisingly, her singing voice is beautiful, high and clear. I tease Shelly that she's going to get a new dad. The comment gets me elbowed in the gut.

My mom doesn't like Mike at all. She interrogates me about him almost every night. How long was he at Brandi's apartment? Was he ever there alone with me and Shelly? Did he talk to me? Touch me?

She's overreacting. Mike seems pretty harmless. He listens to music and messes around with his car's engine down in the parking lot. He spends more time with that car than he does with Brandi. One thing I don't like about Mike is the sour stench of cigarettes on him, but I'm used to that. Even though Mom doesn't smoke, she still reeks of it every night when she gets home from work. Sometimes a sickly sweet smell rolls off Mike. Shelly says it's from something he smokes called pot. Over time, Brandi smells more like that, too.

It turns out I was right. Brandi and Mike elope on a Wednesday night the following spring. In the evening, they show up at my apartment and surprise everyone with the news. Brandi shoves her new gold ring in our faces, grinning. Words slurring, she describes the ceremony.

A red-faced Shelly storms out, interrupting Brandi. We all listen to her feet pound down the concrete steps that separate our apartments. She slams the front door downstairs so hard the noise sets off a car alarm in the parking lot. Mom tells me to go down and check on her.

As I enter her apartment and walk down the narrow hallway toward her room, Shelly's harsh sobs are so loud I hear them through the thin walls. Without knocking, I walk in. She's under the covers, a pillow thrown over her head. I lay down next to her on the pink ruffled bedspread. It's become more bedraggled since the first time I saw it. Broken threads and stains mar its surface. I touch the red splotch next to my arm where Shelly and I spilled nail polish when we were six. Brandi had been screaming mad at us. It doesn't seem that long ago.

Silently, I wrap my arm around Shelly's heaving shoulders. She doesn't like to be talked out of her pain. Over the years, I've learned that trying to use words as comfort at these times turns into an argument. It's like she believes sympathy is an attack on her sadness. Like it's a way of saying she has overreacted. No. Better to let her cry it out.

Eventually, she stills. "I hate him, and I hate *her*," she whispers angrily. "She's so freaking selfish. All my mom thinks about is what she wants. She should ask me what I want. Like ask me before she goes off to marry Mike. It affects me too, so shouldn't I get a say in it? But *no*, whatever makes her happy. I'm an afterthought. She never wanted me in the first place."

Shelly has talked about this fear of being unwanted by her mom before. It all started because of our stupid classmate, Dominic, who lives down the hall. Last year, he told Shelly on the playground that he overheard Brandi say Shelly was a mistake, that she accidentally got knocked up and wished she hadn't had her.

Who knew if it was the truth? Shelly had taken it to heart, though.

At least Dominic wouldn't tell that to anyone else. I made sure of it. I had punched him so hard in the face it chipped his front tooth. The other kids stood in a circle around us, chanting, "Fight, fight, fight," until the principal pulled us apart. As I was being escorted into the front office, I had overheard another student say, "She's crazy." Grinning madly, I was happy, satisfied that no one would mess with Shelly or me again.

My mother had been furious, but I couldn't feel bad about it. This was how my neighborhood worked. If you didn't stand up for yourself, you were asking to be a victim. Once that happened, it was over. All the bullies and predators came out to play with you. I had seen it before, kids' lives ruined because they didn't fight for themselves. It wouldn't be like that for us. I would fight for myself *and* for Shelly, too.

I rub Shelly's shoulder through the blanket. "Just because your mom's married doesn't mean she'll forget you. Maybe things will be even better. She'll have more money because Mike can pay for stuff. I bet you'll get a ton of Christmas presents next year." A twinge of jealousy at that thought. I got two Christmas gifts this year, a book, which I loved, and some new underwear, which I didn't.

Shelly peeks out from under the pillow. Her cheeks are blotchy from crying. "Mom doesn't love me. She just wants Mike."

"I don't think that's true. He always has dirty fingernails. Yours are clean and pretty." I fish under the covers until I find her warm hand. Pulling it out, I look at the chipped pink fingernail polish I had painted on Shelly a few days before. Back when Brandi was still single. At least, we've gotten better about not spilling it.

"Just remember—you are smarter, prettier, kinder, and funnier than Mike is." I tick off my fingers, one for each attribute.

She takes in a shuddering breath. "You think so?"

"I know so."

Her cheeks drying now, she sits up. "My mom doesn't see me that way. I don't even think my mom sees *me* sometimes. She'd rather watch TV or be with Mike."

"Well, then she's nuts, because I'd rather be with you than anyone else." I hug my best friend close. "Don't worry, Shelly. Everything will be okay."

Turns out, things aren't okay. Shelly is moving. Now that Brandi and Mike are married, they want to live closer to Mike's day job. Shelly and I are distraught. We beg Brandi to change her mind but make no headway. I think back to how Shelly called her mom selfish and have to agree.

"You'll still see each other at school, girls. You get to be together there practically every day." Brandi haphazardly throws Shelly's clothing into a crumpled cardboard box. "You can sit together at lunch," she says absently as she frowns at a pair of jeans where Shelly's worn holes in both knees.

"But Mom," whines Shelly, "it's not the same. We hardly have any time to be together at school. The teachers get mad at us when we talk in the hallways, and lunch is only 20 minutes long."

I want to jump in and agree with Shelly but hold back. Brandi isn't my mom, so I'm never sure how much to be involved in these family conversations.

"Besides, what about the weekends? We usually spend all of Saturday and Sunday together. Now we'll live too far away from each other to walk. We won't see each other." Shelly makes the weekend sound like a century of time.

"You can figure out the bus schedule. Maybe there's a bus that goes from here to there," counters Brandi.

This is a losing battle.

I have to give it to Shelly for determination, though. She won't drop it, arguing, "You said last month that we're too young to go on the bus ourselves. You said we couldn't take it down to the aquarium, remember?"

Exasperated, Brandi throws the torn jeans on the floor and stands up. Her voice is tight with anger as she yells at Shelly, "Find a bus or don't. I don't care, but we *are* moving. Stop fighting with me about it."

Brandi rages out of the room, leaving us to finish packing.

11

PAST, LAS VEGAS, NEVADA, AGE 11

Brandi's move leaves me without a daytime babysitter. That familiar worry line in the middle of my mom's forehead makes a nasty reappearance. She sits at the kitchen table late into the night, trusty calculator in hand. Her fingers tap over the keys like it's a genie's lamp and if she rubs it long enough, it will magically produce the money to pay for someone to watch me while she works.

One day, a couple of weeks after Shelly moved, we unload groceries from our rusted hatchback car as we discuss the problem. Mom's been missing work to stay home with me, but she can't keep it up. We need a solution, so I argue that I can stay by myself. I'm 11 now and feel very grown-up. Most of the kids in my apartment building are "latch-key" kids. Shiny silver keys hang on long strings around their necks like badges of honor. They let themselves into their empty apartments after school. All alone, they get their own snacks and do their homework.

Shifting a heavy bag of groceries in her arms, Mom's brows crease with worry. Her eyes dart around, like she's looking for a threat. "Maybe if we lived in a nicer neighborhood and I knew it was safe, you could be by yourself. Did you know that last week Mrs. Rodriguez in the next building over had her apartment broken into? It was at 3:30, just when you would get home from school. Thank goodness she was out when it happened, but can you imagine? What if that was you, Kitten? What would you do? No, I'm sorry, but I can't bear it. Not until you're older."

"Is it because you don't trust me? You think I'll do something stupid?" There's hurt in my voice. I tell my mom everything. I get all As at school and don't get into trouble, except for that one fight with Dominic. Looping my fingers through the handle of the bag I'm holding, I let it swing, hanging down by my thigh.

Mom's tone softens. "No. That isn't it at all. Of course, I trust you. It's everyone else I worry about. You don't know what it's like." Her eyes grow distant. "You haven't learned how awful some people are. How they can look at someone so pure and young as you and want to spoil it. How some people can't stand beauty. They want to make everything as ugly as they feel inside." She's set a bag of groceries down on the hot pavement at our feet so she can use her expressive hands to explain. She's just finished talking when a voice speaks behind us.

"She can stay with me."

We whip around to see our new downstairs neighbor, Mr. Chen, the elderly Chinese gentleman who moved into Brandi's apartment. He has a newspaper in his hands, having retrieved it from his front doorstep. "I can take care of her after school," he repeats calmly, ignoring the identical looks of shock on our faces.

Mr. Chen is slim, shorter than my mom, with gray hair cut close to his scalp. He walks slowly with a cane. Friendly since he moved in beneath us, he's always waving hello and making small talk when we pass him on the way to our car.

But we don't know him.

"Oh no, Mr. Chen. That's kind of you to offer, but I can't take you up on it." Mom's flustered, trying to be polite and hide her surprise that he would suggest such a preposterous idea.

"Really, I don't mind. I'm an old, retired man with a lot of time on my hands. It's understandable, you being cautious, but I promise she'll be safe with me." As evidence, Mr. Chen holds up one bony, wrinkled hand. It's twisted and contracted, trembling with the effort to hold it high.

Point made. There's no way he could overpower me.

Still, other kinds of threats remain. Ones that aren't physical.

My mother resists. "It's too much to ask. I wouldn't be able to pay you. Sometimes I don't come home until late or I work weekends."

"I don't need money," Mr. Chen says. "It would be beneficial for me, too. There are certain things I can't do anymore. Like high-up places I can't dust, for example, or jars I can't open. Tiffany could help me with those things after she finishes her homework. That would be her payment."

Silently, I follow their exchange. I've always had a good feeling about Mr. Chen. A good "vibe," as the kids at school might say. There's something about his eyes, a gentle kindness. Since he moved in, I've heard piano music drifting out his open window and up the stairwell. He plays beautifully, the notes dancing and twining around each other. It might not make perfect sense, but I think someone who makes music that lovely can't possibly be bad.

"It's a good idea." I use my best wheedling voice. "Please, Mom? Can I go to Mr. Chen's when you work?"

Mom looks helplessly between us, Mr. Chen and me. It's a sign of her desperation that her resolve crumbles. "Okay. You can stay with him." She shoots a stern look at me. "You better be on your best behavior, young lady."

"I will, Mama. I will." We hug, ignoring the ice cream melting in the grocery bag at our feet.

12

The next day, I go to Mr. Chen's apartment while my mom works. He makes me take my shoes off and leave them by the doorway on a small shelf. I walk into his place barefoot, the tile floor cool under my feet. Mr. Chen wears what he calls houseshoes, fabric slippers that he pulls on over tall white socks.

Old man footwear.

He catches me eyeing his place curiously, my head whipping around as I take it in. "You can go explore," he says with a soft chuckle.

With that, I'm off, roaming through the apartment. It's strange to be back here, to walk through a place I know so well. Everything is the same but different. Heavy antique wooden furniture with rich upholstery has been placed carefully in each room. On what becomes my favorite chair, there's an embroidered scene of an old-fashioned Chinese warrior in plated armor. He battles a fire-breathing serpent with a spike-tipped pole.

A stand-up piano sits in one corner of the living room. Its warm mahogany wood gleams from careful polishing. The hinged cover of the piano is pushed back, revealing ebony and ivory keys. I run my hand over them lightly, eliciting a tinkling sound that goes from high notes to low.

Shelly's old bedroom is now an office. Bookcases line three of the four walls. They hold thick hardback and paperback books. Some are in Chinese, the symbols trailing down the spines. The only place I've seen this many books before is a library. I run my hands over each one as I walk along, my fingers going bump-bump-bump.

One row has English titles, and I pull a book out at random. I'm startled to see a man staring back. It's a gruesome picture. Half of the man's body has been peeled away in layers to reveal the bones, blood vessels, and muscles beneath. *Atlas of Human Anatomy* by Frank H. Netter, M.D., reads the title and author in bold letters.

The book should disgust me, but it doesn't. I take it to a wooden rocking chair, where I sit and rock slowly, flipping through the pages. Intricate colored drawings of dissected eyes and cut-open hearts capture my imagination. It's crazy how much stuff is crammed into the human body. According to this, each part has its own vital function. I spend so long looking at the book that Mr. Chen comes to check on me. If what I'm reading surprises him, he doesn't show it.

I tilt the cover up for him to see. "What's this? Why do you have it?"

"I was a doctor back in my home country, in Taiwan," he explains.

"I thought you were from China. Is Taiwan in China?" I'm not good at geography, besides having to memorize all 50 states and their capitols last year in school.

Mr. Chen shakes his head. "No. Taiwan is its own country. It's an island, close to the mainland of China."

"Oh, sorry." I had just assumed he was from China. I remind myself not to make those kinds of assumptions in the future.

"It's okay. Most Americans don't know the difference." He sounds resigned to this fact, rather than angry.

"You were a doctor there?" I'm curious to learn more about my new caretaker. Pushing off with my feet, I continue rocking. It soothes me.

"Yes, a cardiologist." Seeing my look of confusion, Mr. Chen adds, "A heart doctor."

Why is he living in a dump like this? I wonder. Doctors usually make a good living. There are lots of fancy suburbs in Vegas. *Why not live in one of those?*

"Which hospital did you work at?" I ask, remembering my mother's lessons in manners.

"At the University Hospital downtown. I was a janitor, though, not a doctor." He winces as he lowers his body into an office chair at his desk.

"Huh? Why would you be a janitor?" My rocking stills as I attempt to figure out this mystery.

"I went to medical school and did my training in Taiwan. My medical license doesn't work in America. None of my degrees apply here, so I took a job where I was most comfortable. At the hospital, a janitor job was all they could give me." He tells me this in a matter-of-fact way. Like it's no big deal that years of hard work got thrown out the window because he crossed an ocean.

I'm furious on his behalf. "What!? Why would they do that to you? Couldn't you do something? Take a test to prove that you're a real doctor?"

"No." His smile is gentle. "It doesn't work that way. I would have to start my medical training all over again. I was too old by then."

When he sees that I'm still upset, he adds, "It's okay, Tiffany. Back home, I had a good career, working for many years. I like to think that I helped people, hopefully saved some lives. I'm grateful for it, but time moves on and things change. You can either change with them or resist and get stuck. I chose to let it all go. To become someone different. Not someone better or worse. Just different, and that's okay."

"Why did you move here, then?" Why would you leave all that money and prestige is what I want to ask, but my mom says it's rude to talk about money. She taught me to ignore different levels of social class because all people and jobs are equally worthy.

That isn't true, though. I've heard Brandi and her friends talking about the men who come to their club and what jobs they hold. Brandi and her cronies scoffed at some careers, but I heard the reverence in their voices when they talked about others. "Doctor, lawyer, judge, executive," they whispered, and I saw the cartoon dollar signs pop up in their eyes.

"I moved for my daughter. I hoped she would have a better life here. She was in high school when we came over. I wanted her to go to an American college, then graduate school. Maybe she could become a doctor like me, if she wanted that." Mr. Chen's expression changes, a subtle shadow in his eyes.

I've never seen anyone visit Mr. Chen. His daughter must live far away. "Where does your daughter go to school now?"

Mr. Chen pauses, and I feel an ominous shift in the air. This isn't new to me, the expectation of disaster. I always have a faint sense that something bad is coming. Now, that feeling is so strong that I know before he even says it.

"She died. Hit by a drunk driver during her second year in college. She got into a great school, UC Berkeley." Mr. Chen's proud of his daughter, even in death.

My imagination takes hold. I picture Mr. Chen's daughter standing beside him, with beautiful midnight hair and soulful eyes. The image is so sad that I begin to cry. With joint-popping effort, Mr. Chen pries himself out of the chair, comes over, and puts an awkward arm around my shoulder.

"I'm sorry. Please don't feel bad." He pats my shoulder gently until my tears dissolve into occasional hiccups.

I wipe my eyes with the back of my hand. "I'm okay."

"Good. Maybe when your mother comes to pick you up tonight, we can skip the part about how I made you cry. Now help me back to the chair. I think my legs are about to collapse." Mr. Chen grimaces.

After jumping up to help him, I flip through the anatomy book on the desk. "Will you teach me?" I ask, looking up from a diagram of the brain.

"Teach you what, dear?"

I like that, being called dear. It makes me feel safe and cherished. *Special.*

Pointing at the anatomy book, I say, "Some of the stuff in this book. Some doctor stuff. The piano too?" I hope Mr. Chen won't think I'm being silly or asking for too much.

"Yes, dear. I can teach you."

13

PRESENT, COLUMBUS, OHIO

The third day of Ethan's training, I had walked into my office to find two desks shoved together in the tight space. Pushed against each other like lovers. Distracted, I didn't notice the new office chair by the doorway. My shin banged into it—hard. Pain flared and with it my temper. "What—what the—," I had stammered, heart slamming furiously in my chest.

Before the expletive left my mouth, Ethan had cut me off, holding up a placating hand. "Washburn insisted. Said Brandon's old office got turned into storage space."

Oh, yeah. That's right.

Hopping around on one foot, I held my throbbing leg until I lost balance and tilted dangerously to the side. Ethan had caught my elbow, steadying me. "It'll be okay," he had said softly, the quiet confidence in his eyes cooling my ire. "We'll make it work." Angry words had died in my throat, and I blinked at him, unsettled. I wasn't used to being soothed.

Now, it's a few weeks into Ethan's training, and we sit, working side-by-side. My backpack is half-open on the floor between us. I bring it with me each day to store my extra pens, notepads, and textbooks. I grab an eraser from the bottom, and it tips over. Most of the backpack's contents spill out. A frustrated huff escapes me, drawing Ethan's attention. Crouching down, I shove the items back in.

Ethan comes over and kneels on the ground next to me. He places books and pens into the backpack. The paperback I'm reading has fallen out. He picks it up and turns it over in his hands, a delighted grin spreading across his face. That's when I notice his mouth quirks a little higher on the right side when he smiles. It's this perfectly imperfect lopsided smile that's so disarming.

I stare at it, mesmerized for a long second. Then I give myself a small shake.

Ugh. What is wrong with me? I'm acting like Amy when she first saw Ethan. Like the rest of the female staff who stop and gawk as he walks by. Not that he looks back at those women. I haven't seen him flirt with anyone…yet.

"Tiffany?"

A minty smell from the gum he chews breezes over me.

"Hmm?" I put the last pencil back in the bag, deliberately ignoring his gleeful smirk.

"What's this?" Ethan holds the book out. It's a cheesy romance, a rom-com, my favorite. A couple kisses passionately on the cover, and a tasseled purple bookmark sticks out. When I see what Ethan has, a blush warms my cheeks. I make a grab for the book, but he moves it just out of reach.

"Give that back," I demand, petulant as a child.

"Not until you tell me about it." He's clearly enjoying himself.

"Geez, Ethan, I think you need to go back to school if you can't recognize a book when you see one," I say sarcastically.

He's not deterred by my snarky tone. "I know it's a book. A romance judging by the cover. Why is it in your backpack?"

I roll my eyes so hard they probably do a somersault in my head. "Because I'm reading it, genius. Back in the days before you came along, I used to get some downtime. I'd read a chapter or two during work. You know, in between patients or at lunch. When I could eat *by myself*." I pin him with a glare and snatch the book away, quickly shoving it into my bag, wanting it out of sight before it can embarrass me further.

Ethan doesn't fall for my insults. He's grown used to my occasional snide remarks. Instead, he goes back to sit in his chair. Pushing with his long legs, he leans the chair back. Under his weight, it tilts dangerously, threatening to tip over and dump him on the floor. Defying gravity, the chair holds. Ethan puts his hands behind his head, lacing his fingers together. "I'm surprised, is all. I hadn't pegged you as a romance reader."

Because I'm such an ice queen.

"I like them, those books." I cross my arms over my chest and tuck in my chin. "They're a nice escape. Totally different from my normal life." Why did I say that? It makes my life sound lacking, which isn't true. I like my quiet existence.

"Different, huh? You don't have a boyfriend?" Now Ethan's the one blushing.

"I have lots of boyfriends."

His head snaps up, eyebrows slashing together.

Laughing at his expression, I clarify. "Book boyfriends, that is." I gesture to the paperback, now safely tucked away in my bag. "Much more reliable than real-life boyfriends. They're there when I need them and go away when I don't."

Ethan taps a finger against his pursed lips and stares at me intently. "When was your last boyfriend?"

A green-eyed boy with a wicked smile flashes through my mind. "It's been a while," I answer vaguely and squirm, not liking how intimate this conversation has gotten. "I do have a significant other at home, though." I make my voice low and suggestive. "He's very clingy, always wanting my attention. He sleeps with me *every* night."

Ethan's eyebrows rise to his hairline.

"It's my cat, Fred. Rescued him my first year of college." I smile, remembering how it had taken an hour and a can of tuna to coax the terrified kitten out of the storm drain. My smile fades as I also remember how much I had identified with the tiny orange cat. After all, we were both orphans.

"He's the *real* love of my life," I tell Ethan, watching his startled expression slowly transform into understanding. "How about you? Any special ladies?" I put a light, teasing tone into my words, happy to redirect the conversation away from myself. In my experience, people enjoy talking about themselves more than they like learning about someone else.

"No girlfriend right now." He's taken his lab coat off and hung it over the back of his chair, leaving him in faded blue scrubs. Ethan's biceps flex as he raises his arms over his head and then back down to his sides, stretching. I could name every rippling muscle in his corded forearms, but I don't.

"Why? Are you hard to please?" The words leave my mouth before I can stop them, curiosity overwhelming my better judgment. I shouldn't care, but it's interesting to learn what makes Ethan tick.

"No. I just know what I want." He has the rubber-band ball in his hands again, throwing it up and catching it.

I rest my chin in my hand and regard him, noting how serious he looks, how he purses his full lips as he concentrates, tracking the movement of the ball through the air. Ethan's a bit of a mystery. He's always calm, cheerful, and confident. Easy to see the surface, but harder to get a glimpse of what lies underneath.

That's the thing about mysteries—they're just begging to be solved.

"What do you want, then?" I ask, all my attention focused on him.

"Someone who will be an equal partner. A woman that I admire. Who knows her own mind and isn't afraid to tell me what she thinks." His answer is quick and sure, like he's given this some thought. He tips his head to the side and pauses, searching for the right words. "I guess I also want someone who likes me as I am. Who believes I'm good enough without having to change or improve. I suppose most people want that. Acceptance."

"Oh." I had expected a flippant response, not this. There he goes again, being open and honest. There's no way I could be that vulnerable. Thrown off, I'm not sure how to respond. "Well," I say, "hope you find her."

His eyes are smoked whiskey today, grazing lightly over my face. A small shiver runs through my body.

With quiet certainty, Ethan says, "Oh, I will."

14

We've been sharing our office for a month when Ethan doesn't show up one morning. He's been working on his own since I finished training him. Now it's 10:00 a.m. and no sign of him. The office is quieter without the hum of both of our computers running. Without our voices blending as we dictate.

I wonder where he is. Should I go ask Dr. Washburn about it? No, that would be weird. I hope something bad hasn't happened. He might have been in a car accident. What if he's lying bleeding on the highway right now? Maybe I should check the Emergency Room? Staring sullenly at Ethan's empty chair with my back to the doorway, I jump when someone loudly clears their throat behind me.

Ethan saunters into the room with a slick, knowing grin. "Hey, Tiffy, what'cha looking at?" His lips twitch with amusement.

I jerk my eyes away from Ethan's desk and narrow them at him. I'm exposed, a kid with her hand caught in the candy jar. "Nothing," I snap, ignoring the guilty feeling at the sharpness of my tone. "And my name is *not* Tiffy."

Ethan's not perturbed. "Really? Because it looked like you were staring at my desk. Like you were missing me."

I scoff. "That shows what a big ego you have, Ethan. I was looking at your desk…and thinking how relieved I am that you aren't here for once."

Ethan stands over my chair and smirks down at me. Suddenly, he bends down to my level, placing his hands on the chair's armrests. He leans over, caging me in. The heat rolling off his body blasts hot as a furnace. His eyes drill into mine, his closeness causing a sudden hitch in my chest.

With soft, slow words, he says, "It's okay for you to miss me, Tiffy. If you were gone, I'd miss you, too." His breath is warm and minty. It breezes over my face like a caress. There's a heaviness growing deep inside, sinking into my core.

Then he's up and away. Sitting down at his desk, Ethan says in a casual voice, as if we had been talking about the weather. "The dentist had a last-minute cancellation, so I went in for a teeth cleaning." He flashes a wolfish smile over to me. "Gotta keep these pearly whites shining."

My flush of embarrassment is followed quickly by fury. He's playing with me, and I hate it. Hate that he caught me with my guard down. Hate that my traitor body reacted with such primal lust at his closeness. All these years of evolution, and I still can't escape that flush of attraction. Ethan knows exactly what he's doing, and it pisses me off.

I snarl at him. "I told you not to call me Tiffy."

Want to see this chapter from Ethan's point of view? Click the link below or scan the QR code to join my newsletter. You'll receive an exclusive bonus chapter from Ethan's perspective that is only available for newsletter subscribers!

HTTPS://TINYURL.COM/ETHAN-BONUS-SCENE

15

gear myself up for a full-blown rant at Ethan, mentally outlining all his flaws, when Dr. Washburn calls, "Tiffany, Ethan, in my office, now."

Geez, can the man for once walk over and talk to us?

With one last death glare toward Ethan, I stalk across the hallway to Dr. Washburn's office. Without even turning, I know Ethan's behind me. I've developed an almost sixth sense to him. We've spent so much time together that my body is tuned to his. I can tell when he is near, just by vibrations in the air.

Dr. Washburn waves us into the room. "Come in, come in."

I spare a glance at Ethan. He looks worried, his eyes darting left and right, like he thinks he's in trouble. I forget he isn't used to Dr. Washburn's frequent summons. I dread the call into this office. It usually means some odious menial task is going to be assigned to us. Last time, Dr. Washburn told me to train Ethan.

Look how that worked out.

"As you know, part of Ethan coming into our residency was an agreement that we would send radiology residents to Highview Hospital in Cleveland to help staff the department there," Dr. Washburn says. "It's difficult to get a resident in the middle of the academic year, so we were lucky to replace Brandon with Ethan." Dr. Washburn nods in Ethan's direction.

I can feel Ethan relax as he realizes he's not in trouble.

Dr. Washburn sees the dark expression on my face. Misinterpreting it for anger over the Cleveland situation, he says, "I'm sure it will be beneficial for you both. The hospital there has a different patient population, which means you'll get exposed to diseases you wouldn't typically see here in Columbus. You'll work with other radiologists who can teach you new skills."

He pauses to blow his runny nose into a tissue, making a loud honking sound. "The hospital will provide you with free meals and housing. They have apartments they rent for situations like this. I want you two to go there next week. You'll set up the rotation. See what they have available and how it can best be used to train our staff. See what needs they have that you can fill."

"W—wait," I stutter. "You want us *both* to go? Together?"

I glance sideways and see the color has drained out of Ethan's face. Looks like he's not too happy with this idea, either. The sting of rejection pokes at me, prying between my ribs and squeezing my heart.

"Yes," answers Dr. Washburn, oblivious to the emotions swirling through the room. "Ethan knows the Cleveland hospital well, so he can help orient you. Tiffany, you understand our residency, so you can determine how we fit into its department. We want this transition to go as smoothly as possible. Once you get everything set up there, we'll send two residents to Cleveland at a time on a rotating basis. I want to instruct the next group on exactly what to expect. It's your job to figure that out."

He drops one last bomb. "As an incentive, if you are successful in this task, I'll give one of you the Resident of the Month award. Ethan, have you heard of it yet?"

Ethan shakes his head no.

"It's a certificate given to one resident in the hospital each month. A generous bonus of $1,000 comes with it. Needless to say, it's very sought after." Another swipe of Kleenex to the tip of his cherry-red nose before he drops the crumpled tissue in the trash can.

"Doesn't some big committee determine the winner?" I ask. I always imagined it as a grand affair, like the gathering of the Continental Congress. White-wigged doctors carefully weigh each candidate's attributes to choose the best one. They all sign the Resident of the Month certificate like it's the Declaration of Independence.

"There is. I'm on that committee. I already told them I'll be awarding it next month." Dr. Washburn folds his hands over his chest and leans back, preening.

Huh. Well, that's disappointing.

So much for an impartial group of men and women handing out the Resident of the Month certificates. This is like finding out that Santa Claus isn't real. "But only one of us can get it?" I clarify, trying to wrap my head around how this will work.

"Yes, you're right. I'll have the medical staff in Cleveland report back to me about how you both perform. That way, I can decide who to give it to."

Why does Dr. Washburn appear so smug when he says that? It's like he enjoys pitting us against each other. Maybe he thinks this is the medical version of the *Hunger Games*. Aggravated, I clench my fists, fingers digging into the soft flesh of my palms.

Unbelievable.

Last month, I lost that award because Ethan ruined my lecture. Now I might lose it again because of him. Dr. Washburn gives us a few more instructions, such as when to arrive at the hospital and where to park. He hands me a badge that will let me enter the hospital.

Dr. Tiffany Hart, Radiology, Highview Hospital.

Ethan still has his old badge from when he used to work there.

Shell-shocked, Ethan and I return to our office.

The X-ray before me swims in and out of focus. I can't concentrate, too busy worrying about Fred The Cat, the only companion who's never left me. Who will take care of him? And what about my beat-up 1990s sedan? Can it make the drive to Cleveland without breaking down? I barely trust the car to travel the couple of blocks between my apartment and the hospital.

Most of all, I'm plotting how to win that award. I desperately need the money for my conference at Disney World. I also want the validation it provides. That certificate is proof that all my striving and sacrifice haven't been in vain.

Ethan's unusually quiet, all his earlier mirth gone.

Finally, I can't take the silence any longer. I spin my chair toward him. "This is your fault," I scold, pointing my finger at him. "I said during your interview this would happen."

Ethan doesn't rise to match my anger. "You're right. I knew this was coming. I just didn't think it would be this soon," he says glumly.

I don't know how to handle this withdrawn version of Ethan. He's usually so outgoing and confident.

He doesn't want to go with me.

Well, that's fine because I don't want to go with him either.

Before I can take it back, the thought flies from my brain and out of my mouth. "You can ask Dr. Washburn for a different resident to go with you. You obviously wish it wasn't me."

Ethan's head snaps up, his eyebrows puckering in confusion. "What? No, that's not it, Tiffy."

"I told you not to call me that." I want to shake him, I'm so annoyed. Shake the defeated look off his stupid, handsome face. Why, of all people, do I have to compete against him? "Ugh," I say, throwing my hands into the air, "I just can't get rid of you, can I?"

"That's right. You're stuck with me." He glares right back, flecks of gold swirling in his amber eyes. There's a certainty to his words. Like he's making a threat…or a promise.

16

Worrying about Fred The Cat weighs me down. In desperation, I text Melanie.

Tiffany: HUGE favor to ask.

Melanie: What's up?

Tiffany: Washburn's sending Ethan and me up to Cleveland for a month to set up the resident exchange program. Need you to watch my cat, Fred. The apartment there doesn't allow pets.

Melanie: Okay. Give me your key, and I'll stop by UR place every day.

Tiffany: Sure? I feel bad asking.

Melanie: It's fine! Love cats. I mean, I think I love them. Haven't spent a lot of time with one yet.

Tiffany: You're making me nervous.

Melanie: No! It'll be fine. Promise.

I pause, wanting to call the whole thing off. But I can't. I have to go to Cleveland, and I can't take Fred The Cat with me. A damp snout bumps my elbow as the feline in question winds around me, purring like a chain saw.

As usual, the cat's presence calms me. I scratch behind his ears and under his chin. Fred tilts his head up with a lazy cat smile.

"Good kitty," I tell him, my voice raspy from disuse. I've had the weekend off, and he's the only living thing I've talked to.

Tiffany: Thanks. I owe you.

Melanie: Drinks when U get back?

I stop typing, fingers hovering over the keys, understanding what Melanie is asking. This is her invitation, yet again, to become friends. Real friends, not just work friends. Do I want that? It's silly, but needing someone to watch Fred The Cat has made me think. Melanie is the *only* person I trust with the job. She's repeatedly shown me I can rely on her. I want to let her know I can do this. Be friends. It's scary, terrifying really, but I'm ready. I square my shoulders and tap out my response.

Tiffany: Deal! I'll buy you two drinks. Seriously, I appreciate it.

Melanie: No problem.

I return to the open suitcase sitting on my bed, along with the pile of clothing that I've picked out to take to Cleveland. When my phone dings, I assume it's Melanie again. My stomach plummets, convinced she's calling to tell me she doesn't want to go to drinks with me, that she can't watch my cat.

Stop it. Not everyone is going to reject you, I chide myself.

It's not Melanie, though. It's something much worse, that strange number again. A sense of foreboding spreads over me as I hold my phone with numb hands, cursing myself for not blocking the number.

No pictures this time. Just one word. Black letters on a white background that reads:

Remember.

I slump down on my bed, barely noticing that I've jostled the stack of neatly folded clothing, toppling it over into a heap. For a long, long time, I stare at that single word with my mind emptied of every thought, every emotion except for one. Dread. That's all I feel. It's a roaring darkness that presses down on my chest, smothering me until I can't take in a breath or let one out.

All the things I've deliberately forgotten. All the things I've hidden. Someone knows about them. But who can it be and what do they want? Are they trying to scare me? Because if so, it's working. Are they trying to blackmail me? I have more student loans than money, so not that. A million different theories spin through my mind, but none make sense. The people I used to know in Las Vegas are long gone. Scattered in the wind.

My legs grow stiff. That's how long I sit there staring at my phone. Finally, I give up searching for answers that refuse to be found. I punch the buttons on my phone and block the number. No more texts. No more being frightened. My heart can't take it. Determined to forget the message, I shove the clothing into my bag, give Fred The Cat one last pat on the head, and leave my apartment.

Time to go to Cleveland.

FRIEND

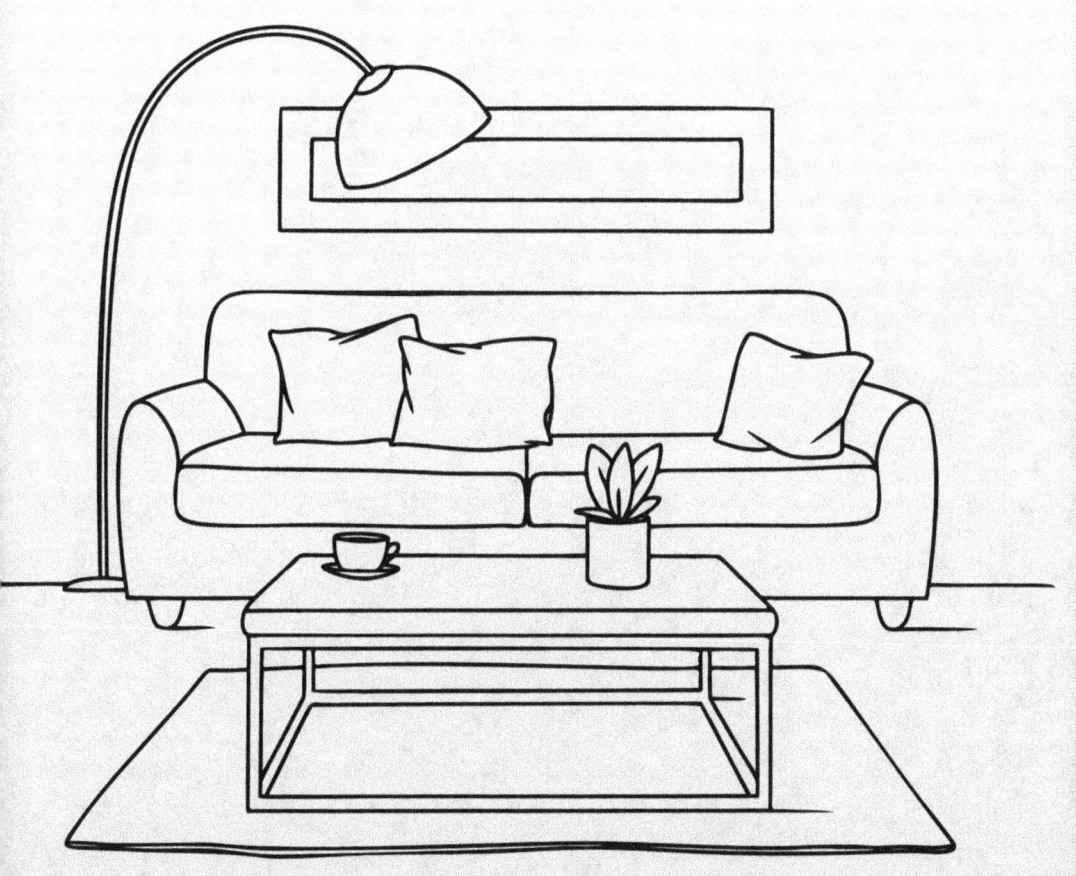

17

PRESENT, CLEVELAND, OHIO

When I arrive in Cleveland, it's past 10:00 at night. A full moon sends its luminous spotlight down to the street, causing light and shadows to dance across the pavement. My old run-down car makes alarming wheezing noises as I pull into the apartment parking lot. It has a chronic oil leak that no mechanic can fix. Once I'm parked, I pop open the hood. I always carry a quart of oil in my trunk. Kicking myself because I forgot to bring a funnel, I carefully pour it into the engine, trying not to drip.

A low voice calls out behind me. "Hey, Tiffy. What're you doing?"

Startled, I jump, and oil splashes onto the engine block.

Why does he always make me spill?

I'm still furious at Ethan about the "missing him" comment when he came back from the dentist and about how unhappy he looked when he learned we were going to Cleveland together. I've also spent a large part of my drive reminding myself that he's my competition for the Resident of the Month award.

"Refilling the oil. My car has a leak," I answer brusquely.

Ethan has parked his SUV right next to mine. It's a sleek black BMW, a limited edition from the looks of it. A swell of jealousy rises and settles in my throat. As if I needed more reasons to dislike him.

Leaning against the front of my car, he watches as I finish up. "Who knew you're so talented? A woman who can name all 206 bones in the body *and* put oil in her car. Not bad." The lopsided smile is back.

Looks like Ethan got over not wanting to be here with me.

He's acting like his usual self now, brash and annoying. It's a relief. He had been unusually quiet that last day at the hospital when we found out we were coming here. I had almost been worried about him.

Done with the oil, I use my full body weight to slam the heavy car hood closed. Ethan jumps back dramatically, pretending like I was going to crush his fingers. I narrow my eyes at him and earn a wide smirk.

"I got the keys to our apartment from the manager. Ready to see it?" Ethan dangles two sets of silver keys from his finger. They glint in the moonlight.

"Wait." I tense. "Did you just say *our* apartment? Like we're sharing one?" An uncomfortable feeling buzzes in my brain. It hadn't occurred to me to think much about the living situation. Dr. Washburn had told us that the hospital was providing complimentary housing, but he hadn't elaborated further.

Ethan's looking at me like I'm crazy. "Yeah. One apartment. You didn't really believe the hospital would pay for two separate ones, did you? You know how cheap they are."

He's right. Hospitals often provide free food and lodging, but at the least possible cost. It's usually run-down buildings and mass-produced food. This will be no exception. It's going to be a long four weeks if I have to live with Ethan.

After gathering my luggage from the trunk, I squint through the bright glare of the parking lot lights to inspect my new residence. It's a two-story concrete building with outside stairwells leading to the upper floors. A couple of bikes are chained to rusted iron railings. For a minute, I have a sense of disorientation, of déjà vu, thinking that I'm looking at my old apartment in Las Vegas. Old instincts kick in, and I glance around, trying to assess if we're in a bad part of town.

"Did you live here when you worked at this hospital?" My eyes rove over my surroundings as I move my suitcase closer, scooting it over with my foot.

"Nah. My place was way nicer than this." Ethan's answer doesn't assuage my fear, and I hesitate.

Ethan grabs both his bag and my small suitcase. "Come on, Tiffy. Last one in is a rotten egg." He takes the metal steps two at a time.

"Stop calling me that." I swear he's trying to irritate me on purpose.

Ethan puts the key in the lock and turns the deadbolt. The door sticks for a second, then pops open with a squeal of protest from its hinges. I hurry as he enters, not wanting to be left outside alone.

Ethan turns on the light switch, revealing the interior of the apartment. It's an open floor plan. A small round dining table is in front of us. Further in the room sits a dated loveseat, coffee table, and bulky television. A low countertop with bar stools separates the living room from the small kitchen, which runs along the right wall. Black appliances reflect the harsh rectangular lights overhead. We walk down the short hallway to explore the rest of the apartment. There's a small bathroom with a shower-tub combo. It has ugly mustard-yellow tile and carpeted floor.

"Yuck. Who puts carpet in a bathroom?" I cringe. Every germ I learned about in microbiology class comes rushing back, and I'm convinced they all live in that carpet.

Ethan shakes his head. "I don't know. That's disgusting."

At the end of the hall are two small bedrooms. They each hold matching furniture—a scarred wooden dresser, a nightstand with a lamp on it, and a twin bed.

"Which one do you want?" He hands over my suitcase.

I choose the one on the right, and Ethan goes left. After I drop the suitcase on the floor, I lay down on the bed without bothering to pull back the bedding. The thin comforter is scratchy beneath me. It's the firmest bed I've ever felt, like lying on top of a boulder.

I groan.

Even though we're separated by a wall, Ethan must hear me, because he yells, "What's wrong?" His voice is so loud it's like he's right there, in the room with me.

"This is the hardest mattress I've ever laid on. It might as well have nails sticking out of it," I answer without raising my voice. I want to see if he can hear if I talk normally. His answering chuckle tells me that he understands just fine.

"Wow. These walls are really thin," I say. I shift, trying and failing to find a comfortable position.

"I know. I can hear you, too."

Rolling onto my side, I face the wall that separates our bedrooms and tease, "Now you'll keep me up all night with your snoring."

"Hey, who said I snored?" he protests from the other room.

"I'm sure you snore with that gigantic head of yours. I wouldn't be surprised if you have sleep apnea." My mouth curves into a smile, which I'm glad he can't see. I'm enjoying this banter a little too much. I need to remember that Ethan is my competition, not my friend.

"No snoring or sleep apnea, but I'll still keep you up at night because listen to this." Through the wall, I hear him bounce on his bed. The bedsprings make a loud, harsh, squeaking noise every time he moves.

"Stop!" I giggle. "That's awful. I give this place a negative one-star rating. Do not recommend." That sends Ethan off in a burst of laughter.

I laugh with him, enjoying how our voices merge and echo, bouncing around the small apartment.

Competition or not, maybe it won't be so bad living here with him.

Curious to see what Ethan's doing, I walk into his room. He's lying on his back in bed with his sneaker-clad feet hanging off the end. He's dejected, full lips turned down in the corners. When he sees me, he says, "I'm not so worried about snoring. I'm more worried about how I'm supposed to sleep in this bed. It's clearly made for a child."

He looks so ridiculous, laying there with his feet dangling, that it makes me laugh even harder.

"Easy for you to find this funny. You fit in your bed. I feel like Gulliver in a bed made for Lilliputians." Ethan squirms. Rolls onto his side and draws his knees up to fit his feet on the mattress. He tucks his hand under his cheek like a child.

"That sucks. I'm sorry," I sympathize.

A moment of silence stretches out as I stand there, watching Ethan. He stills, staring back at me. It occurs to me that it's just us here, the two of us, alone in this apartment. It's oddly intimate.

"Well," I say, clearing my throat, "we should start getting ready to go to sleep. Why don't you use the bathroom first?"

"You sure?" He's already getting up and gathering his things.

"Yeah, I'll go after you're done."

The bathroom door closes with a soft click. Back in my bedroom, I unpack my clothing into the dresser drawers. Although I try not to listen, I hear the toilet flush and the sink faucet running. It's strange, listening to Ethan's evening routine through the wall. Such a private time of the day, usually reserved for solitude or to be shared with a lover. It feels like eavesdropping on a conversation I'm not meant to hear.

Something about it makes me self-conscious. Knowing that in a few minutes, he'll listen to me in the same way. I tell myself to play it cool. There's no need for things to get weird. After what seems like a long time, the door creaks open and Ethan emerges. The clean smell of soap clings to him as he comes to stand in my doorway. "Your turn."

Throwing my towel over my shoulder, I pick up the small bag with all my supplies. I tease, "I think you take longer in the bathroom than I do."

Ethan follows me down the hall. His crooked smile is disarming, and his breath is minty as I brush past. "I have an elaborate system to keep these perfect teeth shining." Cocky, as usual. He leans nonchalantly against the bathroom door frame, tilts his head to the side, and stares at me. His eyes boldly trace the angle of my nose, my jaw, my mouth. I gulp down a swallow, my throat suddenly dry. It's unnerving to have him here, much too close, invading my personal space with all his yummy-smelling manliness.

"Whatever." I roll my eyes, shove him out into the hallway, and shut the door in his pretty face.

Once inside, I pause, staring at Ethan's wet toothbrush and half-squeezed toothpaste next to the sink. The bag holding the rest of his toiletries sits partially open. I resist the urge to peek into it, to see what lotions and potions he uses. He's placed his items in a heap on the left side of the sink, so I neatly arrange my stuff on the right.

Quickly and quietly, I get ready for bed. Toothbrush. Hairbrush. I button up my white pajama shirt to the top and pull the drawstring tight on my matching shorts. I leave the bathroom and stop by Ethan's room to say good night. He's in bed, reading a book titled *The Baseball 100*. White sheets are tucked up under his arms. He's not wearing a shirt, exposing the toned muscles of his upper chest and shoulders.

My eyes dart away, trying not to gawk as I stutter. "I—I just wanted to say good night."

Ethan seems embarrassed at being caught half-naked, mumbling, "Sorry, I can't sleep with a shirt on."

"It's okay." I stare at the wall above his head. "Well, good night."

"Good night, Tiffy." Ethan puts his book face down on the nightstand and turns off his lamp.

Back in my room, I get settled under the covers. Stretching my arm out, I lean over and turn off my bedside lamp. The room plunges into complete and utter darkness. Out of habit, I left the door half open. It's so dim that I can't make out the hallway beyond my door frame. There's just a black pit out there, an abyss. My heartbeat speeds up, a loud thump, thump, thump.

After a moment, I whisper, "It's really dark, isn't it?" I speak so softly that I don't expect Ethan to hear, but his answer is immediate.

His disembodied voice floats back to me. "Do you want me to turn on the bathroom light? I can leave the door open a crack. It'll be like a night-light."

"Do you mind?" I hate to ask, but I don't want to get up. Fears I usually silence have awakened. *Little bird* whispers a voice from my past.

"It's no problem." Fumbling sounds from his room. A sharp curse followed by Ethan announcing, "I'm okay. Just stubbed my toe." Finally, he turns on the bathroom light and partly closes the door, leaving a sliver of yellow to travel up the hallway and illuminate our rooms.

Ethan comes to my bedroom to evaluate the result. He pushes my door all the way open. "What do you think?"

He's standing in my doorway, caught in that golden beam of light. I can't answer for a moment. Too busy staring at him bare-chested in the glow. It highlights his tall, slim frame. The light makes the ridges of his well-defined muscles stand out in sharp contrast. He has a fine smattering of curling chest hair. The drawstring of his pants is undone, and they hang low on his body.

Sharp hipbones peek out on each side with the hollow of his taut stomach between them.

He's stunning.

"Tiffy?" he questions into the silence.

"It's fine. Totally fine. Thanks." My voice is too fast and too high.

"No problem." The details of Ethan's body are lost as he walks back to his room. His bed squeaks when he climbs in. "Good night, Tiffy. I hope you can get some sleep."

"You too. Good night." I calm my racing heart and then, as an afterthought, add, "Try not to snore too loud from your enormous head."

Ethan's laughter is the last thing I hear before I fall asleep.

18

The alarm goes off, jarring me awake. I could swear I fell asleep only a minute ago, but a peek at my clock tells me it's been hours. I yawn and stretch, then remember where I am.

Cleveland. With Ethan.

Cocking my ear, I listen for him. Nothing. He must be awake, though, because the tantalizing smell of coffee wafts through the air. It's the incentive I need to get up. A quick glance at Ethan's bedroom shows that it's empty. The bed has rumpled covers and tangled bed sheets.

Leaving my own neatly made bed, I go to the bathroom. As I brush my teeth and hair, I evaluate my reflection. Tired eyes, pale skin. I hadn't slept well last night, plagued by nightmares. The details of my dreams are hazy, but I can guess what they were about.

Still in my PJs, I leave the bathroom and go down the short hallway. I halt at the entrance to the living room. Ethan's there, dressed in his pajama pants. He has his shirt back on, which makes me relieved and disappointed all at once. Standing on one leg, he slowly kicks his other leg out in front of him. His hands are bent at the level of his chest, palms facing out. In slow motion, he pushes his hands out straight, keeping his palms flexed.

"What on earth are you doing?" I interrupt, unable to process what I'm seeing.

Without pausing, he responds, "I'm doing tai chi. It's how I start every morning."

"You're kidding me." My eyes track his every movement.

"Nope. That move I just did is called High Pat on Horse." Ethan's hands and legs shift slowly, like they're in molasses. "This one is called Carry the Tiger."

"Are you for real right now? You actually know tai chi?" I stare at him with disbelief.

"Totally serious." Ethan lifts his chin. "I also have a black belt in karate, I've won mixed martial arts competitions, and I was an Eagle Scout, which is the highest level in Boy Scouts." He flashes a cocky grin. "See? You're learning all kinds of new things about me today."

I ignore his boasting but must admit there's a certain beauty to his motions. He has a graceful slinkiness that reminds me of Fred The Cat.

"When did you learn all of that?" Watching him makes me extra curious.

"Started martial arts and Boy Scouts when I was in elementary school and stuck with them all the way through high school. I'm *loyal* like that." Ethan shoots an oddly intense look in my direction. "Didn't learn tai chi until college, though."

For a minute, I have a doubling of my vision, seeing the present and the past all at once. I'm standing in Mr. Chen's kitchen, looking out of the sliding glass door, watching him perform these same poses on his tiny concrete balcony. Had I known that it was called tai chi back then? I can't remember.

Bending low, Ethan gracefully extends one leg, balancing easily on the other. Then he rises with his arms outstretched, shifting them slowly up over his head. The pose makes his shirt cling to his chest. Something about how his body ripples with each movement catches my eye. My gaze shifts to watch how his muscles flex and extend in his upper arms.

Staring at Ethan does strange things to my breathing, making it faster and uneven. It's like last night, by the bathroom, and later, when he turned on the light. I'm finding it difficult to look away from him. There's a slow, sweet pulse growing within me, a swell of desire I don't welcome. It alarms me to be so hyperaware of him. I wish I could turn off how my body is responding, just flip it off like a light switch.

To deflect from my arousal, I say stiffly, "Well, it looks silly." I'm surprised when Ethan doesn't rise to my bait. He just raises one eyebrow and gives me a disappointed look. Usually, a barb like that pushes other people away, maintaining my boundaries. I'm not sure how to handle an adversary who refuses to fight.

Ethan continues like I hadn't just been spiteful to him. "How about you? Were you a Girl Scout? I bet you got a lot of badges."

"You'd bet wrong then. I was not a Girl Scout. Afterschool activities weren't exactly a big thing where I'm from unless you count fist fights by the bike racks." I grimace, remembering one particular fight, hearing the crunch of a nose breaking, blood running over swollen knuckles, that flash of green eyes.

"I know how to play the piano a little," I offer. "My neighbor downstairs, Mr. Chen, he taught me when I was a kid. I'm not very good, but I like it. The way music can transport you to far-off places."

Ethan's looking at me with great interest, standing still now. He seems to enjoy finding out these little details about me. Collecting them like seashells on the beach. Putting them into his pocket for later inspection.

It's weird.

I fidget under his scrutiny. "Do I smell coffee?"

"I brought it from home. It's in the kitchen. I also have vanilla creamer so you can make those iced lattes you love." He resumes his routine.

I scrunch my nose and tilt my head, puzzled. "Creamer? But you like your coffee black." In the hospital cafeteria, Ethan never used cream or sugar. Once, I had asked him about it, and he had jokingly told me, "I like my coffee how I like my women, hot and strong." I had laughed when he said it but couldn't stop the blush that had risen to my cheeks.

Ethan's eyes glow warm amber in the morning sunlight. "I do take my coffee black, but *you* don't, so I bought creamer."

Oh.

It's such an unexpectedly thoughtful gesture that I'm tongue-tied, uncertain how to respond. When I enter the kitchen, I'm impressed by the elaborate coffee setup. I didn't see it last night when we first looked around the apartment, so Ethan must have brought it to Cleveland. There's a bag of imported coffee beans, a coffee grinder, and a large espresso machine that takes up most of the counter space.

Humming to myself, I make my coffee and add the creamer from the refrigerator. Pouring it over ice finishes the drink. I take a sip and close my eyes, savoring how the vanilla flavor bursts across my tongue. It's sweet, caffeinated heaven.

Beverage in hand, I return to the living room. There's an old throw pillow, squashed nearly flat, that I move out of the way so I can sit on the lumpy couch. I delicately balance the icy coffee on my thigh. Ethan continues his ritual while I struggle not to notice the sexy way his hair falls over one eye and how firm his butt looks when he bends over.

Jesus, his body is insane.

It occurs to me that there's probably a whole slew of women who would pay good money to sit right here in my spot on this couch and ogle Ethan. How they would love to view the Hot Ethan Clark Show that I'm getting for free. I need to *not* be one of those women.

"Wow. Good coffee and morning entertainment." I try to sound casual, but it's a struggle. "Maybe living with you won't be as bad as I thought."

His smile is slow, like his tai chi. "I like living with you too, Tiffy."

The statement lingers for a few minutes. I shift on the couch, not able to look at him because my heart just gave a weird spasm. There's a new pressure in my chest, one that wasn't there before. I place my hand over my sternum and rub it absently. Maybe I'm having a heart attack. Should I check my blood pressure? Get an EKG?

"Except for when you wake me up with your nightmares," Ethan adds, snapping my attention back to him.

"What?" My whole body tenses.

He continues moving. "Last night. I heard you having a nightmare. I was just about to get up when you stopped. You must have gone back to sleep."

I squeeze my eyes closed, embarrassed. "Sorry."

When I open my eyes, I see Ethan is worried. There's a tightening around his eyes and mouth. "Does that happen often? It sounded pretty bad."

"Yeah. I have a lot of bad dreams. Always have," I admit. "Why? What did I do?"

"Mostly, you thrashed around. You were kind of crying and whimpering." He bends down to touch his toes, surprisingly limber for a man.

"Did I say anything? Talk in my sleep?"

Please, no. Please say I didn't reveal anything.

"No…you didn't really say anything." He ends his tai chi and sits down on the couch next to me.

Good. That's a relief. The more I think about it, the more I hate how Ethan heard me like that. So unguarded. I can't think of any way to gag my dreaming self, though. Hopefully, it won't happen again. I can never predict how bad the dreams will be. They seem to flare up when I'm in an unfamiliar place. It's one reason I didn't want to come to Cleveland.

To change the subject, I say, "We'd better get ready. Want the bathroom first so you can spend hours on your teeth?"

"You know I do." He smiles, showing off those perfect teeth.

19

The apartment is a block from the hospital, close enough that we walk to work. In the light of day, I see that the neighborhood surrounding our apartment isn't as bad as I first thought. The view is typical for Midwest suburbs, one- and two-story brick houses with tall chimneys and wide grassy front yards.

It's fall, and the air is crisp but not yet cold. The leaves have turned, their colors red, brown, and yellow. They dangle, barely holding onto the tree branches, until they lose their grip and flutter to the ground. We walk through that carpet of fallen leaves, our footsteps stirring them as we pass.

When we enter the circular drive that leads to the main entrance, I get my first look at Highview Hospital. It's made of tan brick with a central one-story lobby. Two towers flank the lobby, their tinted windows reflecting the cloudless sky. Silver wheelchairs sit empty by the front doors, waiting for patients.

This hospital is smaller than Mercy Hospital, where I usually work. Hopefully that means it'll be less busy. Ethan and I have an enormous task ahead. Properly setting up a residency exchange program usually takes months, if not years, but Dr. Washburn expects us to do it in four short weeks. The thought of all that work in a brand-new hospital is overwhelming. I'll need to learn the hospital layout, get to know the doctors and nurses, and memorize the hospital's specific protocols.

At least I have Ethan. He already knows his way around this place. It strikes me that we've switched roles. Now he's the one giving the tour, pointing out different areas of the hospital as we walk through. He's so familiar with these halls that it's easy to blindly follow him to the medical education offices. A receptionist has us wait for the medical education director. Dr. Washburn told us to check in with him first. Ethan sits in a tufted brown leather chair in the waiting area, stretching his long legs out and crossing his ankles.

Restless, I pace slowly, trying not to trip over him, and look around at my new surroundings. I stop to put on my glasses and investigate some pictures on a nearby wall. It's a row of portraits of all the medical directors since the opening of the hospital in 1952. Picture after picture of dour old white men.

Typical.

Judging from these photos, you'd think that no women or people of color have ever worked here. I focus on the third picture in the row. Something about the man is vaguely familiar. Squinting at the tiny gold plaque under the picture, I read Nathaniel Clark, M.D., 1998–2001. I stare at the portrait, trying to figure out why it catches my attention. Then the answer comes to me.

"Ethan?"

"Hmm?" He's been quiet, watching me look over the portraits.

I notice he isn't smiling. It's weird to see Ethan without a smile. He has many smiles, from a smart-ass smirk to a shy grin. Blank-faced, he looks different, still handsome but more generic.

It troubles me.

"Is this guy related to you? His last name is Clark, and he kind of looks like you." I point to the picture in question.

"That's my dad. He spent his entire career here. Finally retired three years ago." Ethan stands up and joins me in front of the picture wall.

He points to another photo, much farther down. "My grandfather, my dad's dad. He was one of the founding doctors of this hospital. According to my dad, he was never home. Too busy getting this place up and running. He passed away before I was born." His voice is matter-of-fact, like he's talking about someone else's family.

I move to look at the picture of his grandfather. They must have strong genes on that side of the family. This man has the same features as Ethan and his dad. They all share that full mouth, cleft chin, and dark straight eyebrows.

Even though the picture of his grandfather is black and white, I can tell he has the same golden-brown eyes. Penetrating, they stare out from his face in the gilded picture frame.

With questions swirling through my mind, I turn to look into a younger version of those eyes. Why didn't Ethan mention that his family basically built this hospital? With that history, they must have connections and status in the community. Seems like something most people would bring up. Maybe even brag about.

Just then, Dr. Santos, the medical education director, comes out of his office. "Ethan!" he says warmly. A South-American accent softens the first syllable of the name. He's middle-aged, with dark hair and wire-rimmed glasses.

Ethan smiles widely. "Dr. Santos. Let me introduce my fellow radiology resident—"

"Ah, yes." Dr. Santos turns to me. "This must be Tiffany Hart. So nice to meet you." A dry, cool hand engulfs mine and squeezes gently. "I've known your residency director, Dr. Washburn, for years. Met him at a medical conference when we were just interns. Can you believe it? Time flies by so fast, as they say."

Dr. Santos asks Ethan, "How are you liking Columbus? Is radiology everything you wanted it to be?"

For some reason, the question makes Ethan flush and look sideways at me. "Columbus is great. Going even better than I expected. Thanks for helping me get the spot."

With a rich laugh, Dr. Santos rocks back on his heels. "As if I had any choice. You were always coming by and asking if I had any leads." He addresses me. "Practically every day, this kid was here pestering me to find him a radiology residency position. He was so eager to leave Cleveland."

I feel a pang of sympathy for Ethan. It sounds like he worked hard to leave this hospital, yet here he is—back again.

"Hope he's doing a good job for you all. He promised to work extra hard once he got to Columbus." Dr. Santos looks at me expectantly, and I realize I'm supposed to comment on Ethan's performance.

This would be a perfect moment to sabotage Ethan. I'm sure Dr. Santos is one of the doctors reporting back to Dr. Washburn about our progress. If I want that Resident of the Month award, I need him to think I'm better than Ethan.

Ethan's staring at me like he can read my mind. In my peripheral vision, I see him clench his jaw, bracing for me to say something derogatory.

"He's doing great, sir. We're lucky to have him," I say, looking Dr. Santos right in the eyes.

Ethan relaxes at my words. I'm offended that he didn't have more faith in me. Did he really think I'd throw him under the bus to get that certificate? Once, many years ago, I tried to pull myself up by dragging someone else down. It's a decision I still regret. I won't ever make that mistake again. I will win the award, but I won't do it by dimming Ethan's light.

I'll win by outshining him.

"You both need to sign some quick paperwork, and then you can go to the Radiology Department." Dr. Santos hands us each a stack of papers, which we complete. Then we say good-bye, and Ethan leads me toward the Radiology Department.

"Dr. Santos seems nice," I comment as we walk down one sterile, white-walled corridor after another.

"He is. At the end of every year, he and his partner would have all of us interns and residents over to their house for a barbeque. It was something we all looked forward to. He always treated us with respect, not like some of the other attendings, who act like we're expendable."

I snort. "You mean like Dr. Washburn?" My residency director is always scheming up new ways to shift more responsibilities to the residents so he can work less.

Ethan glances at me. "Yeah, kinda like that."

It takes us forever to reach the Radiology Department. Ethan seems to know everyone in the hospital, and they all want to say hello. Doctors, nurses, and technicians, young and old, stop us in the hallways. I'm regaled by stories about Ethan, like the time he was an intern and slept through a fire alarm. Or when there was a blizzard and the rest of the staff got snowed in, leaving him as the only doctor in the ICU.

"Dr. Clark handled it well," a respiratory technician tells me with pride. "Only had two patients die that night." The burly man claps Ethan on the shoulder so hard that he flinches.

"Oh! That's… good." I try to remember how many ICU patients usually pass away in one day.

An older nurse even tells me about how she remembers Ethan as a small child, coloring in the break room when his dad would bring him to the hospital. The nurse describes how he would sit patiently for hours while his father rounded on patients. "Such a good boy," says the nurse fondly, with a pat on his cheek, which makes Ethan look like he wants to sink into the floor with embarrassment.

By the time we finally get to radiology, my face hurts from all the smiling and nodding I'd been doing. An older radiologist named Dr. Fann shows us around the department and then takes us to our office. When I see the cramped room with two computers side by side, I'm not surprised.

It feels like home.

20

We go through a lengthy tutorial on how to use our new computers. It's noon, and we haven't started our actual work yet. Ethan runs down to the cafeteria to get us lunch. Now that I'm used to his eating habits, I don't comment when he comes back carrying a tray so laden with food that I'm convinced it'll make the table collapse. We eat while we work, sitting at our desks. Ethan offers me a crispy onion ring, but I shake my head no, sticking instead to the French fries that come with my sandwich.

As I chew, I watch Ethan from under my lashes. Everyone has greeted him with enthusiasm today. He's been cheerful and polite in response, but I sense a kind of reserve in him. Like he's holding back a piece of himself here, a part that he usually lets loose in Columbus. It bothers me, this discrepancy.

"They love you here." I say, breaking the silence. "It's like the prodigal son returning, and you've only been gone a couple of months. I'm surprised you ever left. You must love radiology to give up all this adoration."

"I couldn't *wait* to get out of here," he spits out with an intensity I wasn't expecting. "Besides, not everyone likes me."

I raise my eyebrows, questioning.

Ethan says nothing more, going back to his work. The computer screen casts a haunting blue glow over his face.

Interesting.

After a moment, he lets out a frustrated sigh and swivels his chair toward me. "I don't totally understand what we're supposed to be doing here. How exactly are we going to set up this exchange program?"

Since Dr. Washburn gave us the assignment, I've given this a lot of thought. "I have some ideas," I assure him. "How about we break it down based on how advanced we are? For example, a first-year resident who is just starting to learn radiology should focus on reading X-rays and basic stuff. A senior resident can do the more complicated procedures, like angiography with the interventional radiologist."

I pick up a pencil from my desk and fiddle with it, flipping it over my fingers. "The attending radiologists here aren't used to working with us. We need to make sure everyone is on the same page about what they should be doing."

"That sounds good." Ethan leans back in his chair, stretching his legs out and crossing them at the ankles. The tips of his toes brush against mine and a strange zinging sensation runs up my leg.

"We can make a list of cases and procedures for each resident, based on their experience level. I want to pull chapters from our textbooks and from medical journals and give them as required reading for the month. That way, they can learn as they work." I tap the pencil lightly against the table.

"I can't screw this up." Ethan laces his hands behind his head. "I need to make a good impression."

I snap toward him, frowning. "Why? To win the Resident of the Month award?"

"What? No." He gives his head a small shake. "I'm going to help *you* win that."

I scoff, not believing him. "Why would you do that?" How strange would that be? To have someone in my corner for once?

"To be honest, I thought about trying to win it." He straightens, the chair creaking with his movement. "When I left here to move to Columbus, I got a lot of grief. People implied I was selfish. That I had made a commitment and then gone back on it. They made me feel guilty for leaving them shorthanded. It would be nice to get that award. Show them and my family that I made the right decision."

Now Ethan leans forward, his face sincere. "But I don't deserve it as much as you do. You're the smartest, most hard-working resident in that hospital.

You get there early and leave late. You help everyone and don't take credit for it." A pause before he adds, "Also, Melanie told me how you need the money for that Disney World conference."

Melanie, you traitor.

"I don't need your pity." I scowl at him, offended.

"Pity is the last thing I associate with you. I admire you. Everyone does. You work hard and don't care what people think about you."

He says the last part as a compliment, but it makes me feel bad, ashamed. Like I lack the need for mutual respect that normal people crave. "Not everyone can be like you, Ethan," I retort, hurt and angry from his comment. "You don't have to worry what people think because everyone likes you, Mr. Popular. You were probably prom king in high school."

There's silence from him, which means I've hit the mark. "Ha! Knew it," I cry out, victorious. "You really were prom king?"

He nods, eyes on the floor and pink on his cheeks. "Yeah. Senior year." His gaze lifts, something anguished sparking within. "You're wrong, though. I care *too* much about what people think of me. That's why I'm such a people pleaser. I'm trying to convince everyone to like me, so they won't notice all my mistakes, my failures."

Astonished, I whip my head up to meet his eyes. "You? A failure?"

Ethan drops his gaze to stare forlornly at his desk. "I've messed up a lot of things. Let people down. That's why I want to do a good job here. To make up for it and prove I can follow through."

"You didn't fail at that stuff you were telling me about this morning, the Eagle Scout thing and martial arts." Ethan's mournful expression unhinges something in me. I want to soothe his ache. Fix whatever is wrong. Fight whoever made him feel like a failure. I haven't felt this protective since Shelly. It's stupid because this is *Ethan* we're talking about. He doesn't need my help.

My reminder does the trick. Like magic, his gloom lifts and he sits up straight. "I didn't say I mess up *everything* I do. Just some things." He gives me a shy glance. "Now you know and, typical of me, I'm worrying it makes you like me less."

"Who said I liked you to begin with?" I make sure I say it in a teasing voice, not my usual sarcastic one. It's a struggle to be nice, but I like that Ethan showed me his soft underbelly. I could use this moment to take advantage of his vulnerability and push him away. But somehow…I don't want to.

21

My phone buzzes with an incoming text. That sound makes me wince, worrying that it's another frightening message. It's not, though. I haven't had any since I blocked that number. I sigh with relief when I see the message is from Melanie.

> *Melanie: Hey. Fred is great. He let me rub his belly without biting me, so now I'm his BFF.*
>
> *Tiffany: Wow. You're a cat whisperer.*
>
> *Melanie: How's Cleveland? What's the hospital like?*
>
> *Tiffany: Smaller. Older. People are nice. Their computers were running on outdated software. No IT here, so I updated their system. It was easy, but they were super-impressed. Acted like I was a genius. Lol!*

I pause my texting to smile at the memory. The entire radiology staff is still raving about how much quicker their computers are working. It was a big win for me. I'm hoping my success gets reported back to Dr. Washburn and helps my chances of becoming resident of the month.

> *Melanie: Good! Will U finish setting up the program in time? I know U were worried.*

Tiffany: Not sure. It's a lot, but we're trying.

Melanie: How's Ethan?

Tiffany: OMG. You will never believe this. We live together!!

Melanie: Shut up! What?

Tiffany: Yep. Have our own rooms but share everything else.

Melanie: Wow. How's that?

Tiffany: Not as bad as I thought. So far...

22

Glass shattering. Bloody knuckles. Little bird. Let me go.

I wake from my nightmares with a scream buried in the back of my throat. Heart pounding, I sit up in bed and search the darkness but find nothing. The monsters aren't here. They aren't under this bed or in this closet. My monsters left me years ago, abandoned me. I miss them, even though I shouldn't. Now, the only monster left is the one that lives under my own skin.

These thoughts are too dark. I push out of bed and check the clock. It's past 2:00 a.m. Following the band of light that flows down the hallway, I go to the bathroom and splash water on my face. My neck cracks as I bend it from side to side, trying to ease my tension. It's no use. I'm wired. Adrenaline surges through my body. No way I'm going back to sleep anytime soon.

Hoping fresh air will calm me, I head to the narrow balcony off our living room. The sliding glass door makes a loud grating sound as I open it. I squeeze through and step outside. Two cheap plastic chairs are crammed into the space. I choose one and sit, shivering, as the cold seat touches the bare skin of my legs. The evening breeze is chillier than I expected. I should have brought a blanket with me, but I'm too tired and lazy to go back inside and get one. Instead, I pull my knees up to my chest and wrap my arms around them.

When the door shudders open behind me, I jump and let out a startled yelp.

Ethan steps onto the balcony. He's put his shirt back on. With barely a glance my way, he takes the other chair. "Nightmares again?" he asks, staring at the cracked pavement of the parking lot below us.

I sigh. "Yes. Did I wake you?"

"You did, but it's okay. I'm not a great sleeper either." Ethan puts his feet up on the rusted metal railing and pushes, tilting his chair back until only its back legs are on the balcony floor. The plastic groans as he flexes and relaxes his feet, rocking.

I wrap my arms even tighter around my legs. "Sorry."

"Honestly, it's fine. Want to talk about it?"

"No." The last thing I need is to describe my dreams to Ethan. No matter how scared I am, I'll never tell him.

There's a beat of silence and then he stands up and leaves. After a minute, he's back. Wordlessly, he drops a blanket over my legs. I tuck it in around me and crane my neck to see him next to me. He holds a beer bottle in one hand and has another tucked under his arm. There's a pop as he twists off the cap. Ethan hands me the drink and then opens his own before sitting back down. I snuggle into the blanket, grateful for its warmth.

He takes several swigs in a row, then presses the glass bottle against his right knee with a quiet groan that sounds like he's in pain.

"You okay?" I take a sip of my drink. It fizzes in my mouth before I swallow.

"Yeah. Old baseball injury. It's going to rain tomorrow. I can always tell because it makes my knee ache." He rubs the cold beer along the outside edge of his leg.

"You played baseball?" This is the first time I've heard him mention it, but I remember all the times I've seen him play catch with my ball of rubber bands.

"I was *obsessed* with baseball. Had a scholarship for it in college." His voice deepens, becomes bitter. "Thought I was going to be in the major leagues until I busted my knee sliding into home. I collided with the catcher and tore a bunch of ligaments. It took two surgeries to fix it. That's how I learned tai chi. It was part of my rehab."

I peer through the darkness, trying to see his expression, but the shadows hide it. "That's awful, Ethan. I'm sorry. I assumed you always wanted to be a doctor, since your parents are."

Now his voice has the detached tone it had when he showed me the pictures of his dad and grandfather. "My parents wanted me to go into medicine.

They made me take all the premed classes as a fallback in case baseball didn't work out. I humored them. Took the classes and did okay. Never thought I'd actually use it." His chuckle has a hollow sound. "Turns out they were right. My baseball career ended, and I went to medical school." Another gulp from his bottle. "Want to know the crazy part?"

"What?" My heart aches for Ethan, for the dreams he lost.

"In the end, my parents were right. All those years resisting, trying to prove I was different from them." He shakes his head. "Turns out I like being a doctor. It's nice, knowing I can make a difference, that I make someone's life better. Maybe it's weird, but I feel most at home in the hospital."

I think back to the story I heard earlier today from Dr. Santos. Of Ethan, desperate to leave Highview Hospital. "But not *this* hospital? It seems like you wanted to leave Cleveland?"

His gaze is heavy on me. "You're right. I don't want to be here."

"Why?" I tuck the blanket tighter around my bare feet.

He peers up at the stars like he's looking for inspiration, a way to piece his ideas into words. "Too much pressure. My dad and grandfather are legends. Both of them dedicated their whole lives to this hospital, spent more hours here than they did at home with us. My older brother did his internship and residency here. He's a genius, getting his Ph.D. now, because apparently the M.D. wasn't enough to satisfy him." I can't see Ethan roll his eyes, but it's there in his words.

"I'm proud of them, but there isn't anything left for me. Everything I do gets compared to them, and I hate that. Do you know how many times I heard I was 'just like my father' or 'just like my brother'? Or, even worse, people saying how my brother was better or smarter than me?" He rips a hand through his hair, mussing it, and lets out an aggravated sigh. "I don't want to be like them. I want to be like myself. I want to be a good doctor but still have a life outside of work." The words rush out, one chasing after another.

I remember how pale Ethan was when Dr. Washburn told him we were coming to Cleveland. At the time, I thought it was because he didn't want to be here with me, but now I see the real reason. It wasn't about me at all. It was about him returning to this place so full of memories. A place where he feels trapped by other people's expectations of who he should be.

His voice drops low, whispered like he's telling me a secret. "I told you how I didn't get into radiology on my first try."

"I remember." It's dreadful, seeing how this one moment of failure pains him. It's a bruise he can't help poking. Sometimes things hurt so badly it almost feels good to relive them.

"Everyone here in the hospital knew about it. I don't know who told them. Maybe my dad? He was still working back then. The thing is, no one was mean. They were nice, which made it even worse. All those pitying looks." He pauses and shakes his head forlornly. "If I stay here, I'll always be that little kid who followed my dad around."

Ethan's conflict surprises me. I had only thought of the positives that came from a family legacy. It hadn't occurred to me that there are drawbacks too. I can certainly understand the urge to escape your past and run to someplace new.

For a fleeting second, I think of telling him about the mistakes I've made. Then he might feel less alone in his imperfections. But that's a ridiculous thought. A treacherous one. The less he knows about my past, the better. Right now, he's looking at me like someone he respects. How quickly that would change if he knew the truth.

Instead, I reach over and put my hand on his forearm. We both still, staring down with equal surprise to where our bodies connect. I give his arm a light squeeze. "It's okay, Ethan. You can be whoever you want. You don't have to let anyone else choose a path for you. Success doesn't come from a place." A picture of a concrete apartment in a sun-drenched desert plays through my mind. "Success comes from inside yourself."

His voice is lighter when he speaks again. "That's one thing I admire about you, Tiffy. Your confidence."

"Me?" I touch my hand to my chest in disbelief. I've never thought of myself as confident.

Stubborn? *Yes.*

Confident? *No.*

"You know exactly where you're going. I've floundered and flailed around, trying to find my way, but you're like an arrow shot straight at your target. I've never seen you hesitate." Ethan's bottle clinks as he sets it on the ground.

"I've gone off course before," I correct him. "And most of the time, I don't feel confident. I keep thinking someone is going to take away everything I've built. Like they're going to come and say I'm not a real doctor. That's why I always wear my lab coat and badge. I put on my glasses, sometimes even when I don't need them. I've found that people listen to me more if I'm a stereotype of what a doctor should look like."

A small chuckle from him. "I'm not sure the glasses are working. They just make you look like a sexy librarian. I know what you mean, though. There's a lot of pressure to meet people's preconceived ideas."

I agree with Ethan, although now I'm hung up on his librarian comment. Does he really see me that way? Surely not. I try hard not to project sexy. I don't want that kind of attention. It can be dangerous.

CRUSH

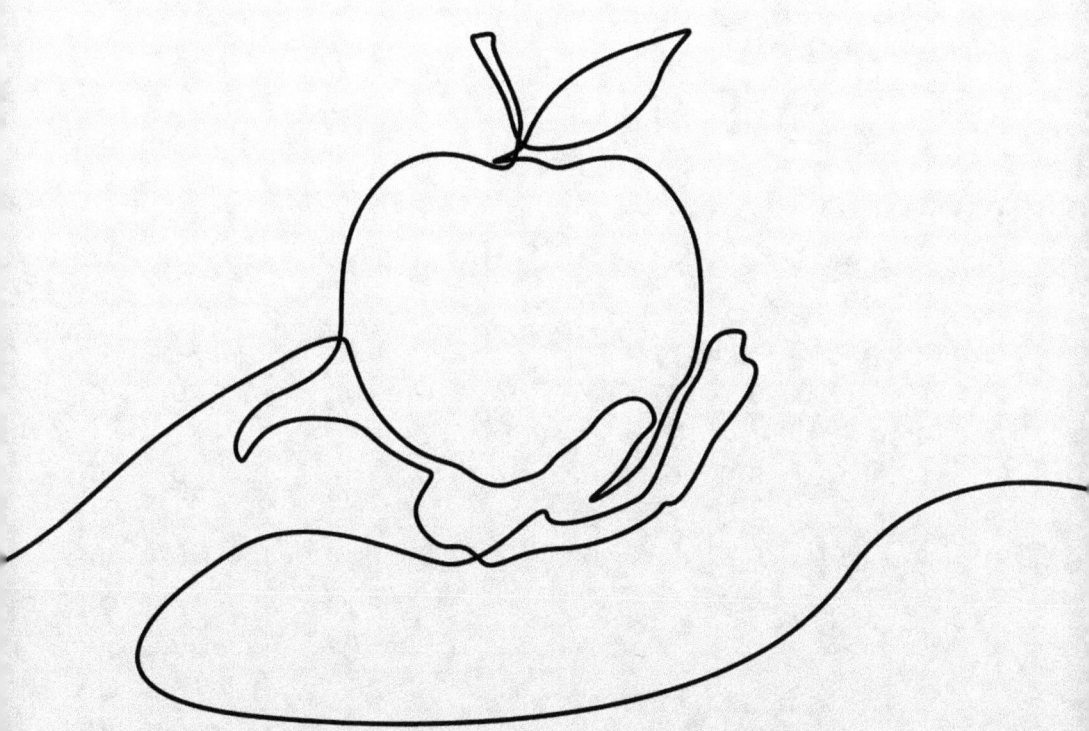

23

PAST, LAS VEGAS, NEVADA, AGE 16

"You sexy little brat," the boy says, emphasizing the word "sexy."

I don't know his name, but I've seen him watching me. His hungry eyes have followed me as I crossed the schoolyard. I'm used to men staring from a distance now. Ever since I grew boobs and a butt, it's been that way.

Never as close as this, though.

"Think you're so much better than the rest of us, don't ya?" His body presses me against the cinder-block wall behind my high-school auditorium. Rough skin scratches my cheeks as he tries to force his mouth against mine. Whipping my face side-to-side, I avoid his lips. His breath smells like cigarettes and onions. It mingles with the smell of trash from the dumpster next to us. I swear I'll never eat onions again after this.

Inpatient hands tug at my shirt. "Always got your nose in a book. Think you're so smart." He looks at me with a mixture of lust and hate.

Hands raised, I try to fight him, but he easily bats me away. I don't know what I did to deserve this. Keeping a low profile at school, I spend time either in the classroom or the library, always studying hard. I was on my way to return a book when he grabbed me and pulled me back here. He's a teenager like me, but big and strong.

My cries for help are lost in the sound of our struggle.

Years ago, my mom warned me about this. When I turned 13 and my figure started to develop, she had stood behind me and picked up a lock of my bright copper hair. "You're getting so pretty, Kitten," Mom had said in her saddest voice as she ran the strands through her fingers.

I had been confused. Wasn't it a good thing to be pretty? Shelly and I spent hours searching through women's magazines, trying to decipher the minuscule differences that made one woman more beautiful than another. We tried to replicate those models, stealing our mother's makeup and jewelry. Giggling as we put lipstick on each other, exclaiming, "You're *gorgeous*, darling," in fake British accents.

Now my mom was telling me it was a bad thing to be attractive. "People…men…are going to look at you in a certain way. You'll have to be careful. Don't draw attention to yourself."

It's this conversation that comes back to me as the sun-warmed bricks burn my skin. The boy finally gets his hand under my shirt, ripping it in the process. My shouts for help get louder. Reality sets in. This is happening, and I need to stop it *right now*.

Just when I've lost hope, a shape moving so fast it blurs crashes into the boy. The attacker is pushed off and falls to the rough pavement. The sudden movement unleashes my sobs. I should get up and run away, but my legs aren't responding. My whole body trembles so hard that my teeth chatter.

I watch helplessly at the scene unfolding in front of me. That blur turns out to be another kid from school. Even though I've never talked to him before, I know this one's name. It's Raphael, but everyone calls him Rafe. He's hard to miss, with languid cat green eyes and a devilish grin. He never walks or runs, just casually saunters around our campus like he owns the place.

Moving faster than I've ever seen from him, Rafe pins the boy down on the ground and sits on top of him. He presses his face close to the kid beneath him and sneers, "You little piece of trash. What do you think you're doing?"

The boy squirms, not bothering to answer what is clearly a hypothetical question. A look of pure rage has replaced Rafe's usual sardonic expression. When Rafe's fist comes out of nowhere and pistons into the kid's face, both the boy and I whimper at the resounding crack of his nose breaking. Blood gushes down his face, a river of red.

Rafe leans in closer. "If you ever, and I mean *ever*, so much as look her way again…" Rafe's blood-stained hand grabs the front of the kid's shirt. He pulls the boy's head up and slams it back on the pavement. "I'm going to mess you up real bad." Another head slam into the ground. "Understand?" The boy is still conscious enough to nod.

Rafe stands, pulling the kid with him. He gives the boy one last shake, sending arms and legs flapping like a rag doll. Then he sets him on his feet and shoves him away. "Get out of here. I don't want to see your face again. If I do, I'm gonna bust it wide open."

The boy scurries off, leaving a trail of blood behind him.

With the boy gone, Rafe turns to me. I lie huddled on the ground, knees tucked into my chest and arms wrapped around the sides of my head like I'm practicing for an earthquake drill. When he kneels in front of me, I flinch backward, slamming into the wall behind me. My sobbing intensifies.

Rafe holds up a hand and ever so slowly moves it closer to pat me gently on the knee. The kind of comforting pat a grandmother might give you if you fell off your bike.

"You're okay. Tiffany, isn't it?"

I nod my head miserably. I didn't think he knew my name.

Now that the fight is over, Rafe loses some of his bluster. He looks around like he wants someone else to deal with my hysteria. Finding no help nearby, he sighs and gathers me up in his arms, holding me like a child. It's comforting. I rest my head against his hard chest, all modesty forgotten in my trauma.

When he starts to walk toward the school, carrying me, I panic at the thought of everyone seeing me like this, tear-soaked with torn clothing. It won't be hard to figure out what happened. I don't want to be known as the girl who got attacked. The weak girl who couldn't fight for herself. I clutch Rafe's shirt and mouth the word "no."

He changes course, understanding my silent plea, and heads for the parking lot. We end up at a beat-up truck, the color so sun-faded that it's impossible to tell if it was once gray or silver. It's been lifted. Aftermarket bright red shocks are visible in the wheel wells.

Juggling me awkwardly in his arms, Rafe kicks open the passenger door and gently hoists me up into the seat. I sit high in the tall truck, easily seeing over the tops of the surrounding cars. He moves around the vehicle and climbs into the driver's seat. Once settled inside, he turns on the engine. Latin rap music blasts out of the speakers, so loud that I clap my hands over my ears. He quickly dials down the volume until the music is a faint hum in the background, and I lower my hands.

The air conditioner gives a rattling gasp and turns on. Hot air bursts into my face and then slowly turns cold. It's soothing, the air drying the sweat from my hairline. I'm still crying. It's like a dam has burst open inside of me, and I can't plug it up.

A silence settles between us. He looks out his window, giving me privacy to pull myself together. Eventually, I calm down enough to speak. "Thanks for helping me." It's a whisper as light as a feather.

He nods in acknowledgment. "That guy's a jerk. He won't try it again," he says gruffly. "You should be fine. If he, or anyone else, bothers you, just come to me, and I'll take care of it."

I wonder what kind of power Rafe has that he can make these promises with such confidence. Maybe I should be more suspicious, but I believe he can deliver the justice he's threatening.

"Okay," I agree. "You're Rafe, right?"

Emerald eyes turn my way, and my breath catches. It's likely residue from my earlier adrenaline rush, but everything appears extra sharp and in focus. Like I've developed some kind of super vision. I can see the ebony stubble on his cheek. The slight chapping of his lips. Rafe's not classically good-looking. The artist who drew him was too heavy-handed for that, but he possesses a dark beauty. He exudes magnetism, and I feel its pull.

"Yeah, that's me." His voice is deep, a man's voice in a teenager's body.

I try to remember if he's one or two grades ahead of me. The silence settles again, making me self-conscious. Maybe he doesn't want me here? Should I leave? About to crack open the door and escape, I stop when Rafe asks, "Where do you live? I'll drive you home."

Caught off guard, I stutter, "Oh, it—it's okay. I can catch the bus."

When I look down at my watch, I realize it's later in the afternoon than I thought. The public transit I usually take home has already come and gone. The next bus won't arrive for another 45 minutes and by that time Mr. Chen will start to worry.

Although I've outgrown the need for a babysitter, most days I still go to Mr. Chen's after school. He's kept his promise and teaches me piano and interesting medical facts. When I get stuck doing my homework, Mr. Chen is there to help. He's good company, quietly puttering around while I work.

I consider calling my mom to come pick me up but decide against it. She's home sleeping, preparing for a night shift. Mom has looked extra tired recently, dark circles under her eyes and her normally pale skin so translucent I can trace the branching river of veins at her temples.

Not wanting to bother my mother or Mr. Chen, my decision becomes easy. "Yeah. I could use the ride." I give Rafe my address and directions to the apartment.

Without another word, he puts the truck into gear. It's a stick shift, so his hand grasps the ball-tipped stick between us. He rests his palm loosely on top, with his hand so close he could touch my knee with the slightest movement. Watching that hand out of the corner of my eye, I'm not sure if I want it closer or farther away.

Red still stains the creases of Rafe's knuckles. I assumed it was from the boy, but now I see fresh blood oozing. He must have broken the skin.

"You're hurt," I exclaim, dismayed. My body lurches toward him, wanting to examine his hand.

Rafe rears back at my sudden movement, shying away. "It's nothing." His jaw clenches.

"But you're bleeding," I protest.

His laugh is deep and harsh. "Trust me. I've had worse." His eyes scan the road ahead like he's ready for danger to jump out at any moment.

Uncomfortable with the quiet between us, I resort to small talk. After all, Rafe isn't filling the air with chatter. "Do you like school?" I ask and then wince. *What kind of lame question was that? Who am I? Someone's nosy great aunt at Christmas?*

This earns me a response, at least. An ironic smile crosses his face briefly before falling away. It was a nice smile while it lasted, white teeth against dark skin. "It's okay. Guess we have to go, right? It's good for business."

What does that mean? He's certainly not selling textbooks. It might be better to stay ignorant about what "business" Rafe does. Before I know it, we're pulling into my complex. He parks in front of my building, angling his truck so it takes up several parking spots at once. The engine is still running. The heavy door screeches as I wrench it open. I free fall to the ground, landing on my feet so hard that the impact reverberates up my legs. At least I don't stumble or embarrass myself. When I stand on my toes to peer over the seat, Rafe is looking down at me, his face impassive.

"Well, thanks again…for saving me." It sounds lame to my ears, but I can't come up with something better.

"No problem." He leans over and grabs the handle of the door that I've left open. Just before he pulls it closed, he says, "Try to stay out of trouble."

Then he's gone, leaving a plume of exhaust behind.

Something changes at school after that day. The boys no longer look at me. Instead, they deliberately look away. It's so obvious that I decide to test its limits. I place myself right in front of a guy from my gym class and stare into his face. He's terrified. Quickly averting his eyes, he rushes past, almost knocking me over in his haste.

Rafe must have said something. That's all I can figure out. I can't imagine the kid who attacked me told anyone. It wouldn't look good for him to admit his crime or how he got beaten. Besides, I hadn't seen him since the attack. Maybe he fled. Or maybe something happened to him?

No, it must have been Rafe. It's like he's claimed me, left his mark. Told everyone I was off limits.

So much for getting invited to homecoming this year.

A few days later, I approach him at school, hoping to say thank you again and to ask what he said to the other boys. As we pass each other in the hallway, I call out Rafe's name. He looks straight at me, so I know he heard, but he walks right past, his face an emotionless mask. I'm open-mouthed, watching his retreating back.

Fine.

We aren't speaking to each other. Message received. Act like we don't know each other.

I can do that.

24

I start to watch Rafe. Before I hardly noticed him, but now I can't stop staring. Each morning, I scan the crowd, searching for a pair of green eyes. A strange tightening in my chest intensifies bit by bit until I see him, then it relaxes and I can finally breathe.

Many days, Rafe doesn't show up at school, which sends me into a panicked spiral of thoughts. *Where is he? Is he okay? Did something bad happen to him?*

A day or two later, he always turns back up. His sudden reappearance like a rabbit pulled out of a magician's hat doesn't help my anxiety. Often, he sports fading black eyes, scraped hands, and bruises in the shape of fingerprints on his arms.

Who hurt him? Is he in a gang? Does his father beat him?

It's probably drugs. Selling them or taking them. I favor selling because I've never seen Rafe act like he's high. He's always carefully controlled, never exuberant or carefree. He doesn't seem like he would enjoy the loss of inhibition that comes from being wasted.

I want to ask Shelly about it, but something holds me back. Things have been strained between us lately. She's changed. Now when she comes over to spend the night, dark eyeliner and maroon lipstick appear on the bathroom counter. Often she's moody, wanting to be alone and listen to music with her headphones on. I don't like it. Shelly has a new set of friends in the apartment complex where she lives with Mike and Brandi. Maybe these girls are influencing her. For so long, I've been Shelly's best friend, but now I'm not sure if I still hold that title.

It's lonely to not share these secret thoughts with Shelly. I want to tell her how I believe I owe Rafe a life debt. He saved me once. Now I daydream I'll save him too. In my fantasies, I'm strong, battling evil forces to protect him. I imagine that seeing my goodness will change him. He'll see the error of his violent ways and convert to a peaceful life with me. I'm convinced he has a soft heart under that bleak exterior. After all, he saved me, didn't he?

My dreams always end with us together in a pretty house surrounded by a white picket fence, something I've only seen on TV. That house is the exact opposite of the utilitarian concrete apartment I live in. That house is an oasis, a mirage in the desert of Las Vegas.

Rafe is my first crush.

25

PRESENT, CLEVELAND, OHIO

It's Sunday, our first day off since we started working in Cleveland. Ethan's just finished his workout when I walk out of my bedroom, dressed and jabbing gold earrings into my earlobes.

A phone rings and I tense, worrying that it's another threatening text message. Which is stupid since I already blocked that number. It isn't my phone buzzing, though. It's Ethan's. Wiping sweat off his neck with a towel, he answers it.

"Hello." A puzzled smile lights up his face, and I'm suddenly curious to know who's on the other end. Is it a woman? The green stab of jealousy is so unexpected that I sit down on the couch with a thump.

Ethan's talking into the phone. "What? Now?!" His voice rises, and his eyes widen in alarm. They snap to our front door like he expects marauding pirates to smash through at any moment. His tension transfers to me so quickly that I jump when heavy pounding sounds on the door.

"Ethan!" a deep voice booms from outside. "Open up."

My eyes race back to Ethan to gauge his reaction. I'm not sure if I should answer the door or go hide in my closet. The hand holding the phone has dropped to his side, and he's staring up at the ceiling like he's having a long, private conversation with God.

The knocking continues. I half rise from the couch, ready to move toward the door, but Ethan beats me there. His hand on the doorknob, he sighs and looks over at me. "It's my brother. Just…ignore most of what he says." With that vague statement hanging in the air, Ethan swings the door wide.

A hurricane of a man sweeps into the room, already talking a mile a minute. I instantly see the family resemblance. Same light brown eyes, cleft chin, and full mouth. This man's eyebrows arch higher, and he's shorter and stockier than Ethan. If Ethan is rectangular in shape, then this man is more of a square.

"Geez, bro, why'd you take so long? Were you naked? Watching porn?" His baritone voice fills our tiny apartment. He half-embraces, half–choke holds Ethan into something resembling a bear hug. "I've been standing out there forev—."

When the man's eyes land on me, all movement stops as his mouth falls open in a perfect O. Ethan uses the pause to extract himself out of his brother's arms, prying them off his neck. His brother snaps back into motion, an enormous grin stretching his face.

"Well, well, well, who do we have here?" he asks, stepping closer to where I stand by the couch. After a quick glance up and down, he turns an approving gaze to Ethan.

I frown, offended, about to respond harshly, when Ethan interjects. "Curt, this is Tiffany, my fellow resident. We're here *working* together." I don't miss the emphasis he places on the word.

Ethan's amber eyes meet mine. He sends me a silent plea to calm down. I take in a deep breath, puff out my cheeks, and blow it out. I kick my foot at the threadbare carpet a couple of times and try to control my indignation.

"Tiffany," Ethan continues his introduction, "this is my brother Curtis, Curt for short."

I nod my hello, undecided if I like this sibling of Ethan's.

Curt looks disappointed to find out I'm only Ethan's co-worker. He shakes his head sadly and tells me, "They didn't have residents as pretty as you when I was doing neurosurgery. I can tell you that much."

"Oh…thanks?" I say awkwardly, unused to flattery. "Wait. Aren't you training in California?" I furrow my brow, confused by his sudden appearance.

"Yeah. I'm at Stanford, getting my Ph.D. in regenerative medicine. I've got a few days off, so I came back to surprise my little bro and visit some old friends." He shoots a warm, affectionate glance at Ethan.

"Oh!" My hand flutters up to my chest as I turn to Ethan. "I can't believe it never occurred to me before. Your parents live here. Are you going to go visit them? Are they coming here, too?" The thought of meeting Ethan's parents sparks a minor panic in me.

Curt answers for Ethan. "Our folks are away on a cruise. Mediterranean. It'll last the entire month." He turns to Ethan. "You timed that one on purpose, huh?" He jabs Ethan in the ribs with a sharp elbow. It must hurt because Ethan winces.

Curt tells me, "Our dad can be a bit of a—" He leaves the rest unsaid, with me trying unsuccessfully to fill in that blank.

"It's just a coincidence that I'm here while they're gone," Ethan grunts out, body curling around his wounded ribs.

I glance between the brothers, noting their similarities and differences. "How far apart are you? In age, I mean."

Again, Curt jumps in. "A year and a half. But in elementary school, they moved me forward a grade. So we were always two grades apart." He claps a heavy hand on Ethan's shoulder and squeezes hard. "Ethan told you I'm wicked smart, right? Got into Mensa when I was six," he brags, pushing out his broad chest and throwing his shoulders back.

Surprised, I look to Ethan for confirmation, who rolls his eyes and nods. "It's annoyingly true. He really did test in when he was six."

I do a double take when I see Curt's wide smirk. It's a mirror image of the one Ethan uses to annoy me.

Curtis flings an arm around Ethan's shoulder, dragging Ethan down to his height. "I'm a good big brother, though. Did Ethan ever tell you about the time I kicked a kid's butt for him?" Delight spreads over his face when I shake my head no.

He continues his story, keeping a firm hold on Ethan, who has begun to squirm. "It was all on account of Ethan's braces and his neck gear." Curtis chortles. "Remember that, Ethan? How you had to wear that neck thing for an entire year? Gosh darn ugly contraption." Ethan is turning a shade similar to a ripe tomato. "Anyway, I'm allowed to tease Ethan about it because I had to live with his skinny butt. But when another kid in his class started heckling him, calling him metal mouth and stuff like that, I stepped in. I gave the kid a reason to get braces of his own. Popped him right in the old kisser." He waves a fist in the air.

It's probably not the right response, but I laugh at the story, which makes Curtis beam and earns me a betrayed look from Ethan.

"That's funny. I did a similar thing in school. Cracked a kid's tooth for tormenting my friend," I admit without thinking, picturing Dominic crying as the principal pulled me off him.

Two sets of amber eyes blink at me in astonishment.

"What?" I say defensively. "It's okay when a guy does it, but not a girl?"

Curtis eases up on Ethan, allowing him to stand to his full height. Rubbing his neck, a sheepish Ethan admits, "That is kind of a double standard."

"Damn right it is!" proclaims Curt. He points to me. "You give 'em heck whenever you want, Red."

Guess both brothers like to assign nicknames. I sigh inwardly, already knowing that I'm going to be called Red for the rest of the day.

The brothers continue to razz each other, alternating which one of them tells me silly stories about their childhood. They're trying to outdo each other. Ethan ranges from looking mortified to happy. Curtis is hysterical, saying the most outrageous things. They've soon got me in stitches, laughing until my stomach hurts. I'm enjoying this brotherly interaction. As an only child, I've never seen siblings this close up before. It's a bit like watching lion cubs play with each other at the zoo. The same rough housing with a hint of aggression.

We order in for lunch, play card games, and put on a baseball game to watch with beers in our hands. I contemplate giving the men time alone, but they automatically include me in every activity. It's nice, being enveloped in their familiarity and treated almost like a family member.

At one point, when Ethan goes to the bathroom, Curtis tells me in a hushed voice, "You guys are lucky to have Ethan in your residency. He's supersmart and hardworking. Plus, he's nice, too nice if you ask me."

Curt stares at me with calculating eyes, begging me to contradict him. I don't. He continues, "When Ethan left here, several nurses cried. Real tears. Of course, some of them just wanted in his pants. Lucky guy got the better looks, but still, they didn't want him to leave. That's how great he is."

"Do you ever tell Ethan those things?" I whisper back, hoping Ethan will stay in the bathroom and not interrupt this conversation. "The nice things you just said about him, about being smart and hardworking." I add, "Not the getting in his pants part." Given the flatness of Ethan's voice when he talks about his family, I have the impression he doesn't always feel like he belongs with them. If he knew how Curt views him, it might heal some of that hurt.

Curtis snorts in response. "You're clearly an only child, Red. Brothers don't do that. We don't say sweet stuff to each other unless Mom makes us." I'm about to convince him that's stupid when Ethan returns and we drop it.

At twilight, Curtis offers to play catch with Ethan at the park down the street.

"Why?" Ethan scoffs. "You know I'm way better than you."

"Yes." Curtis sends exaggerated head nods and eye flicks toward me. He lowers his voice. "I'm trying to make you look good in front of the beautiful lady, you dummy."

I act like I'm not listening and pretend I don't notice the blush that spreads over Ethan's cheeks.

In a songlike voice, Curt calls, "You're coming along, too. Right, Red?"

I'm already reaching for my sneakers. "I wouldn't miss it."

Both men smile at me, so pleased it makes me freeze. I'm not used to making people this happy. It feels a bit like responsibility.

Ethan produces a worn baseball and glove that I've never seen before. When I give him a questioning squint, he shrugs, trying, and failing, to appear casual. "Keep it in the bottom of my suitcase."

We are off to the park. As the sun sets behind them, blazing warm red, pink, and yellow, the brothers throw the ball back and forth. I watch them from the bleachers, holding a hand up to shade my eyes.

Curtis was right. Ethan looks good with the ball and glove in his hand. A gentle wind tugs on his clothing, pressing his shirt tight against his muscular chest. His biceps flex, straining his sleeve, as he sends the ball with near-perfect accuracy across the field. It's a little hard not to stare. When I pry my eyes away and see Curtis watching me with a sly grin, my cheeks warm and I know they're turning the same color as the sunset.

26

Bloody knuckles, running down the Las Vegas Strip, a coffin lowered into the ground.

I had hoped that after such a nice day with the Clark brothers the nightmares would leave me alone.

No such luck.

I peel myself out of bed, sticky with fear and sweat. My breathing is labored. Running from my dream demons is exhausting, as always. I grab the blanket from the end of my bed and wind it around myself.

When I get to the balcony, I'm surprised to see Ethan outside. I'm usually the first one out, then he follows. As I sit, he hands me a beer already opened. A shaft of light bleeds through the curtains to illuminate him. I watch his Adam's apple bob as he takes a drink from his own bottle. I swallow thickly, although I haven't touched my beer yet.

"It must be nice, having your brother visit. He's such a character." I smile, remembering some of Curtis's most entertaining stories and jokes. I also remember when Curtis said good-bye earlier tonight, how he had dragged me in for a rough hug and quietly whispered in my ear, "Keep an eye on Ethan for me. Make sure he's okay." As I stepped back, our eyes had met, and I had nodded in agreement.

Now, I doubt it was smart to make that promise. Who am I to be responsible for Ethan's well-being? I've proven myself to be an unreliable friend in the past.

"It was good to see him." Ethan's voice is slow, thoughtful. "We drive each other crazy sometimes, but we love each other too."

I wait, sensing there's more.

"A lot of his personality is an act. When he was younger, he would try to cover up his intelligence, didn't want to be left out or made fun of. Back when he was 13, he would spend hours in the bathroom. My parents were in a fit about it, all awkward, not sure what to do. You know what they thought he was up to in there." An embarrassed twitch of his eyes to mine. I nod, my cheeks heating. "I decided to expose Curt, couldn't wait to humiliate him. Next time he was in the bathroom, I flung open the door. Very dramatic, as 11-year-olds tend to be. Guess what I found out?"

Ethan doesn't wait for my response. "He was in there reading Shakespeare's works. Like the entirety of Shakespeare's plays and sonnets. The whole thing. I laughed and laughed, but Curtis was mad I blew his cover. Took one of those heavy books and hit me over the head. My mom had to come and drag us apart."

We both chuckle, laughter leaking out of us into the cool, dark air. A street light flickers, blinking on, off, and on again in the parking lot below.

After a minute, once the light stays solidly on, Ethan continues. "It wasn't all fun, though. Curtis can be over the top. He make some people angry. It's true that he fought the kid for me, but much more often I had to get *him* out of fights. Play peacemaker."

"You think that's one reason you're a people pleaser?" I question, thinking about how easygoing Ethan is. How he gets along with everyone. "Trying to keep people happy? Not fighting?"

His sigh wisps over to me, resignation on the wind. "Probably."

"He told me he thinks you're too nice sometimes," I confess, curious to see how Ethan responds.

"Curt's not the first person to say that." His shoulders slump, and his head rotates slowly to me. "What do you think?" he asks in a quiet voice. "*Am* I too nice?"

I sip my beer, contemplating. It's not that he uses his kindness as a mask. Ethan's not fake. It's more like he wears it as armor. It keeps things on the surface so you don't dig too deep. But ever since I met him, and especially here in the darkness of this balcony, he's given me glimpses of his more private side. I like it, seeing him sometimes flawed and sometimes flawless. "I think it's nice that you're so nice."

The slow curve of his cheek lets me know I've made him smile. He's so handsome when he smiles like that, open and radiant. I think back to how he looked playing baseball in the park today. How his body moved with catlike grace, all his rippling muscles. His expression of unadulterated joy.

Scrunching my nose, I search for something real to tell him, to make him happy. He deserves that. "It's rare to find someone kind and…trustworthy."

My words straighten Ethan's spine. Confident again, he swigs back his beer. His eyes reflect the light from the window as he whispers, "Thanks."

But I'm not really listening, too busy wondering why I used *that* word.

Trustworthy.

Do I believe it? Could I ever trust Ethan enough to let him in? To show him the full me? I search myself but find the answer keeps shifting.

Yes, no, yes.

Flickering like the light beneath us.

27

I throw myself into work. For every radiology case that Ethan reads, I read two. When a technician comes to get us for a procedure, I'm the first to jump up and volunteer. I introduce myself to each doctor and staff member until their names all blur together.

After lunch, at the end of our second week in Cleveland, I corner Dr. Santos in the hallway outside of the medical education office. He pushes his glasses up his nose with his index finger. "Yes, Tiffany? How can I help you?"

"Some of the medical students said they haven't had much formal training in radiology." My hands are buried deep in the pockets of my white lab coat, so he can't see how I ball my fingers into nervous fists. "I could put together a series of lectures to give during their noon educational conferences. One would be about chest X-ray interpretation, the next would be about abdominal X-rays, and so on. I'd cover the topics they would encounter as interns or on call shifts. That kind of thing. What do you think?" Holding my breath, I anxiously wait for his answer.

"Why, that's a wonderful idea." Dr. Santos claps his hands together and beams at me. "The medical students would enjoy that. Our interns and residents would get a lot out of that as well." He lowers his voice conspiratorially. "Just between you and me, some interns have a hard time telling the difference between pneumonia and congestive heart failure. They could use a refresher."

I roll up on the balls of my feet, excited by his enthusiasm. "Really? That's great. I'll work on the lectures this weekend and should be able to give them early next week." Already planning the presentation in my head, I know exactly which slides to put in and the best way to arrange them.

About to walk away, I remember my promise not to undermine Ethan. "Dr. Santos." He looks at me expectantly. "Ethan could give a couple of lectures, too. He's learned enough of the basics that he can teach them."

"It would be excellent to have Ethan on board. I'm sure he's been well prepared since he had you as his teacher." Dr. Santos drops a quick wink before he leaves.

As I walk back to the Radiology Department, I'm glowing from his praise. I'm coming for you, Resident of the Month award.

My phone dings, and I tug it out of my pocket.

> *Melanie: Sorry it took me so long to respond. Was watching an old Caleb Lawson movie. That man is FINE. Even my boyfriend thinks he's hot.*
>
> *Tiffany: Agree. Superhot. Heard he's dating a doctor, but probably just a rumor.*
>
> *Melanie: Lucky woman. Did you know Fred snores? No idea cats did that. It's adorable.*
>
> *Tiffany: I know! Sounds like an old man.*
>
> *Melanie: How R U doing?*
>
> *Tiffany: Good. On track to finish. One week left.*
>
> *Melanie: Awesome. Congrats!*
>
> *Melanie: Ethan??*
>
> *Tiffany: Not so bad. He lets me pick out what to watch on TV. I'm torturing him with Hallmark Channel Christmas movies. Holiday Star is my favorite. He complains, but I think he secretly likes it.*
>
> *Melanie: No way. My boyfriend and I take turns picking out what to watch.*

Tiffany: He's not as bad as I thought. Next patient ready. Gotta run. Kiss Fred for me.

Melanie: I will. See U in a week.

Tiffany: See you.

28

"Tiffy...Tiffy...Tiffy! Wake up!"

Someone's shaking me awake. Half-asleep, I flail out, smacking into a hard chest. There's a loud curse, and my arms are pinned. I panic and struggle. "Get off me! What are you doing?"

"Calm down," says a deep voice, close to my head. "You're having a nightmare."

I sit up with a start. Heart pounding. Mouth dry. When I wipe my cheeks, my fingers come away wet. I've been crying in my sleep again.

Large, warm hands are wrapped around my upper arms. I stare at them stupidly, then slowly trace them back to their owner. It's Ethan, sitting on the side of my bed. Holding onto me like he's scared I might fall off a cliff if he lets go. He waits until the haze of the nightmare leaves my eyes and only then releases me.

I had been running in my dream, my white dress billowing around my ankles, the fabric so long that it tripped me as I ran and ran and ran. I looked back to see what was chasing me. It was a man in a mask, the elegant kind like you might find in Venice, Italy. In my nightmare, those empty eye holes had glowed red, lit from within. Awash in fear and guilt, I had screamed in terror…

That's when Ethan woke me.

"What happened?" My voice is scratchy from sleep. I know the answer to my question but don't want to admit it.

Ethan tiredly rubs his face with both hands. He looks exhausted, dark circles forming under his eyes. "You were having a nightmare…again."

It's our third week in Cleveland, and I've interrupted his sleep every single night with my nightmares. All the other nights, the dreams have led me out onto the balcony. Often, Ethan has joined me there. It's much easier talking to him in the darkness, where he can't see my face. We've continued to share pieces of ourselves with each other. Pretty pieces and ugly ones, too.

This is the first time he's come into my bedroom. I must have really frightened him. Lit by the light from the bathroom, Ethan looks at me curiously and asks the same question that he's asked every night. "What are the dreams about?"

I give the same answer I've offered each night. "I don't remember."

It's a lie.

He closes his eyes for so long that I think he's fallen asleep sitting up. He opens them and pins me with a hard stare. "You're going to be the death of me, aren't you?"

I assume Ethan means I'm going to kill him with sleep deprivation, which is a bit melodramatic. "You can go back to bed now. I'm sorry I woke you." I truly feel bad about it. Ethan shouldn't have to pay for my sins.

"Are you sure you'll be okay?" His eyebrows knit together.

I try for a breezy response. "I'll be fine. Seriously."

After he goes back to his room, it takes us both a long time to go back to sleep. Lying in bed, I listen to the squeaking of Ethan's bedsprings as he tosses and turns. It's over an hour before his room becomes silent.

It takes even longer for me to succumb that night. When I finally do, the bad dreams chase me into the darkness.

29

Even though I'm groggy from a lack of sleep, the next day work goes smoothly. Ethan and I have been taking turns giving radiology lectures at the noon conferences. We're making great strides in setting up the radiology exchange program. Only a few more tasks need to be completed before we go back to Columbus. The thought of leaving makes my chest ache ever so slightly. It's been nice having someone around all the time. Less lonely.

Toward the end of the day, Ethan tells me that he's going to run some errands before coming back to our apartment. I nod distractedly, focusing on a complex MRI case and only half-listening. Afterward, I realize I should have told him to get more vanilla creamer. I'm almost out.

It feels odd to come home to an empty apartment. I've gotten used to a routine with Ethan. Usually, we walk home and change out of our work clothing. Ethan gives me a few moments alone while I catch up on emails or read. He seems to understand that I need some quiet time to reset.

We order dinner or make something simple together. Ethan is a better cook, so I'm his sous-chef and mostly chop vegetables. After dinner, Ethan pretends to fight with me about what to watch on TV until he eventually gives in, and we settle down to see the show I picked. Then it's off to the bathroom, where Ethan spends an abnormally long time on his teeth, and finally to bed.

Now, barefoot in the kitchen, I busy myself tidying up while I listen for his return. Not much later, the front door opens and closes. I listen as Ethan's foot falls walk to his bedroom. Thirsty, I go to the refrigerator to pick out a drink.

Ethan comes into the room. He's changed into the more comfortable T-shirt and athletic shorts that he likes to wear outside the hospital. The shirt hugs the gentle curve of his muscular chest and shoulders. He places a new bottle of my creamer in the refrigerator, reaching past me, his arm gently brushing my shoulder. The heat from his body transfers to mine. His scent of clean soap, laundry, and mint gum washes over me. I'm suddenly aware of how close he is. I could reach out and touch him, press my finger into the cleft in his chin…but I don't.

"Thanks for getting that," I say, a bit breathless.

"No problem." He leans against the closed refrigerator door, only inches away, and gives me his most charming smile. I can't look away from it. Something in me melts, just a little.

Ethan casually asks, "What do you want for dinner?" There's a subtle shift in my mind, a resettling in my bones just from those simple words. When you live with someone, that question is as common as breathing. It hits me, what I've been ignoring these past few weeks. *This* is what it feels like to share your day. To let another person in. To let your decisions be influenced by someone else's wishes and desires. To stop being selfish and instead live a life ruled by compromise.

What do you want for dinner? my mother asks.

What do you want for dinner? Mr. Chen asks.

It's been so long that I almost forgot what this felt like, this sense of being more than just myself. It makes me catch my breath. There's a slight tremor in my voice as I answer, "I'm fine with whatever you want."

We fall into our pattern. Dinner, TV, bedtime.

That's when I find out the real reason for Ethan's shopping trip.

I'm in the bathroom, washing my face, when I hear a loud motorlike whooshing. I go to investigate. Ethan's in the center of his bedroom, kneeling on the ground and overseeing the inflation of an air mattress. As the air blows into it, the mattress unfolds like the petals of a flower. Behind him, there's a newly opened box that reads "queen air mattresses—superior comfort" on the side.

When he sees me, he stands up and, with a flourish of his arms, says a proud, "Ta-da!"

"What's this?" I ask suspiciously.

He explains, yelling over the noise of the mattress inflating, "I'm tired of sleeping with my feet hanging off the end of the bed."

"But we only have a couple more days here." I raise my hands with my palms to the ceiling in a "what the heck?" gesture.

"I know. I know. I should have bought it earlier, but it didn't occur to me until now. Figure I can use it whenever I come up here or when I go camping. It'll be a good investment in the long run." He's clearly overjoyed with his purchase, humming happily as he puts clean sheets and blankets on it.

In the bathroom, I finish getting ready for bed. Afterward, I stop by his room to say good night. Ethan's in his new bed with his shirt off, looking quite comfortable.

"Tiffy." He hesitates for a fraction of a second and then continues, "Do you want to sleep here? Maybe you won't have any nightmares. There's room for us both." He lifts one corner of the comforter invitingly.

I stiffen, blood rushing to my face. "No. I'm fine in my own bed. Thanks."

"I promise not to ravish you." He wiggles his eyebrows in a comedic suggestive way.

It eases my tension and makes me giggle. I sober and shake my head. "No, really. I can't. Thanks for the offer, though."

"Okay. Your loss." Pulling the covers up to his chin, he closes his eyes. "Good night."

Back in my room, the hallway bathroom light spills golden rays across the floor. Silence from Ethan's room. I'm guessing he's already sleeping. How nice it must be to fall asleep like you don't have a care in the world. Ethan has the restful sleep of an unburdened conscience.

I haven't slept like that since I was 18.

I toss off my covers, shiver, and then pull them back on. Blinking in the dimly lit room, I practice deep breathing. It seems to take hours, but eventually I tumble into the darkness.

The nightmares find me.

Hiding, running. Not one, but two coffins sink into the ground.

With a start, I jerk upright, the dream sound of sirens still ringing in my ears. My heart thunders in my chest, and sweat cools on my skin. Shadows ooze down the walls. They crawl across the floor, reaching for me with razor claws. If I go back to sleep, I'll drop right back into that same nightmare. I'll sink into it like my pockets are filled with rocks and I've walked into the surf.

I don't want to be alone with those terrors. On tip toes, I creep into Ethan's room, hoping he's awake. It's nights like this when we end up on the balcony. But his new bed must be working too well because he's asleep, lying on his side facing the door. His handsome face is slack and peaceful.

You're on your own, kid, I tell myself. I'm about to leave when Ethan's eyes crack open. He stares at me dreamily.

"Sorry. I had a nightmare. It—" I start to explain, but he cuts me off.

"Shhh...." His long arm reaches out, and his hand beckons. "Come here."

I pause and take a step out the door, considering. Apprehension, fear, and a need for something I can't quite define...comfort or companionship, maybe...war within me.

Fear wins.

"I can't." My voice is gravelly, a whisper trailing off as I turn to go.

Ethan's next words stop me in my tracks. They sound a lot like begging. "Please, Tiffy. Please. I'm *so* tired. We need to sleep."

Okay. Fine.

But I won't like it.

With great reluctance, I walk over to the inflatable mattress. Ethan scoots over far to the left side so I can claim my spot on the right. I lay down, and with a wide sweep of his arms Ethan throws the blanket up into the air. It falls, opening like a parachute to settle over both of us.

Turning my back to him, I shrink into myself, timid now that we're here together. Ethan moves a little closer, and I tense, but he doesn't touch me. His breath is warm on the back of my neck as he sighs out a sleepy, "Sweet dreams, Tiffy."

I predict that it will take me a long time to fall asleep with him next to me, but it doesn't. Within minutes, my eyes flutter shut, and I slide into a deep, dreamless slumber.

Free of monsters.

30

Ethan's muscled shoulder pillows my head when I wake. Scared to move, I freeze and try not to let all of my weight fall onto him, but still I'm pressed up against his chest. We must have moved into this position sometime during the night. Like our sleeping bodies couldn't bear to be apart.

Slowly, coming fully awake, my senses kick in. I smell the clean, soapy scent of his skin so close to my face. There's the gentle whoosh of his breath above me. In my sleep, I've kicked one leg over him, wrapping my foot around to hook under his calf.

Just as my muscles start to twitch from holding still, Ethan stirs. He wiggles and stretches himself awake. After yawning, his voice floats down to me. "Hey, Tiffy. You up?"

I nod silently, embarrassed to be caught with him this way, with our bodies all tangled together.

A vibration under my ear signals a chuckle. "How'd you sleep? No one put a pea under this mattress, I hope?"

He's so relaxed and nonchalant. Like this happens every day. Two co-workers cuddled together on an air mattress in some random apartment in Cleveland. It isn't something I've ever done before. The few short-term flings I've had over the years didn't involve much cuddling. Just free dinners and unsatisfactory sex.

Ethan's waiting for my answer, so I set aside my embarrassment. "Honestly? I slept great." It's the truth. Most mornings I wake up with a fatigue-induced headache because I sleep so badly, but this morning the pain is miraculously gone. I feel truly rested for once.

"See?" His voice rises a notch, ringing with pride. "What did I tell you? Air mattress to the rescue."

I pull away to sit up. "Don't get too big of a head over it. It's not like you solved world hunger."

"Oh, it *is* a big deal," he boasts with a wide, cocky grin. "I got Dr. Tiffany Hart to sleep peacefully through the night. I'm expecting the Nobel Peace Prize committee to call me at any moment."

Ethan's lean muscled arms cross behind his head, propping it up so he can see me better. His hair sticks up at odd angles, mussed from sleep. A dark stubble has grown along his jaw overnight. Gold flecks glitter in his amber eyes.

He's devastatingly handsome.

The open way he grins up at me sparks something wild in my heart. Maybe he feels it too because that grin slides into a softer smile, more tender and intimate. The world slows down. There's a stillness shimmering between us. A tension that wasn't there a minute before. My body is hollow, filled only with longing. My foolish heart skips a beat, then, to make up for it, pounds twice as hard.

Ethan's full lips part. The soft exhale of his breath caresses my face, as his eyes dilate and fix on mine. I'm leaning toward him, a flower orienting to the sun. Inches away, I freeze. We stay like that, in suspended animation, for a long, long minute. Staring into each other's eyes.

Then I flee.

Unnerved by his beauty and the feelings brewing inside me, I quickly crawl out of bed onto the cold floor. I need to get away from him before I do something stupid. "Gonna go brush my teeth," I mumble and run.

In the bathroom, the mirror reveals my overly bright eyes and disheveled hair. "Get a grip," I whisper fiercely to my reflection, not recognizing the woman who stares back.

31

Ethan's already up and out of his bedroom by the time I come back from the bathroom. A fact I'm thankful for. Now that I'm fully awake, reality hits like a sucker punch. My body flushes, remembering everything that happened. I can't believe I went to him like that. It was my choice, to crawl into bed with him. My own weakness. For years, I've prided myself on not needing anyone. Letting Ethan see me vulnerable last night, letting him help, makes me feel foolish and defenseless.

Even worse, it was the best night of sleep I've had in months, maybe years. And the thing this morning—that moment when my lips were inches from his—I don't even want to think about that.

Praying Ethan is gone so I won't have to face him, I pad on quiet feet down the hallway and peer around the corner. There he is, doing those ridiculous tai chi moves in the living room. There's no avoiding him. I psych myself up to say something mean and sarcastic. It's time to push him away, to remind him I'm a rose with sharp prickly thorns.

"Hey, Karate Kid. How's wax on and wax off going this morning?" I say in my best snarky tone as I flounce toward the kitchen.

Ethan raises his eyebrows at my performance. "Good morning to you, too, Sleeping Beauty."

The word "beauty" bounces around my head like a ping-pong ball as I enter the kitchen and skid to a stop. My iced coffee sits on the counter waiting for me. Ethan must have prepared it. I take a tentative sip. It's perfect, exactly how I like it. The wind gets taken out of my spiteful sails. It's possible I'm overreacting a bit. After all, it was only sleep. It's not like we had sex or anything. And we didn't *actually* kiss.

Cautiously, I carry my iced coffee into the living room and sit on the couch. Ethan ignores me, but he doesn't seem angry, just like he's concentrating. His eyes stay focused on some far-off middle distance. I drink my delicious coffee and watch him move gracefully through the poses. His muscles bunch and loosen as he bends. When he lifts his hands above his head during one pose, his shirt rides up, exposing a slice of smooth tan skin.

Don't look.

Finished with his routine, Ethan plops down on the couch next to me. The cushion bows under his weight, creating a hollow. Leaning back, I try not to topple into him. Can't get too close this morning, not when the sensation of his body against mine is so fresh in my mind. Ethan furrows his brow, like he's thinking hard about something.

Here it comes. We're going to have an awkward conversation about last night.

"When the next group of residents come up to Cleveland, we should have them start on the ultrasound biopsy rotation, not CAT biopsy. What do you think?" He looks at me questioningly.

"Oh…okay?" I stammer out, surprised.

"Great." Ethan rubs his hands together. "That's settled. What about the call shifts? The next group will have to take some call. Do you think three a week is too many?"

I say hesitantly, "I think that's fine?"

"What about textbooks? Which ones should we recommend they bring? Do we need to determine a minimum number of cases that they should read each day? Should we prerecord a video explaining the curriculum we set up? Dr. Fann might give one educational lecture a week if we ask him." Ethan is all business, firing off ideas left and right.

That's when I realize we aren't going to talk about the nightmares or the sleeping arrangement or the maybe-almost kiss. Ethan's doing this on purpose, talking about work to spare me. Get me back in my comfort zone.

The wall I've built against him crumbles, tiny pieces of brick and mortar falling to the ground. My muscles relax as I search him, looking for something to fear and finding nothing. There must be a strange expression on my face because Ethan halts mid-sentence and cocks his head to the side. "What?" he asks softly. "Why are you looking at me like that?"

How can I explain my swirling thoughts in my mind? I'm not used to this sensation, this strange rush of gratitude. Not used to feeling safe. I'm wonderstruck, so I shake my head and say, "Tell me again how you think the call shift should work."

* * *

Later that day, we're back in the hospital. Work is busy, but we're making great progress. We're almost done setting up the resident exchange. Ethan acts like nothing strange happened between us, making it easy to fall back into our routine.

Until nighttime, that is.

When it's time to say good night, Ethan looks pointedly at me and gently pats the empty spot on the air mattress next to him. Like last night, he's deliberately positioned himself on the far left side of the bed, leaving the right wide open.

I begin to argue but stop. Getting a good sleep last night was life-changing. It washed away years of exhaustion. It's tempting to feel that way again. To have the world sharp and colorful, not dulled by fatigue like usual. With a sigh of defeat, I shuffle over and climb in next to him. I turn my back to him and don't complain when he pulls me close and spoons me with one arm loosely thrown over my waist.

"Good night, Sleeping Beauty." The soft whisper in my ear sends an infinitesimal shiver through my body. Too small, hopefully, for Ethan to notice. I fall asleep quickly. If I dream, I don't remember it in the morning. We sleep together like this for our last couple of nights in Cleveland.

It's the best sleep of my life.

32

Our cars are packed. The apartment has been cleared out. The trash can is full of the half-eaten grocery items we couldn't quite finish. It was hard for me to throw away food like that. I still remember back in college and medical school when I was broke and alone, surviving on ramen and water.

Ethan searches through the apartment once more to make sure we haven't left anything behind. Waiting next to my car, I watch him lock the apartment door for the last time. He jogs easily down the stairs to me. I drop my set of keys into his outstretched hand. He'll return both sets to the apartment manager before he leaves for Columbus.

An awkward silence settles.

"Well, thanks for being a good housemate." He hesitates, seemingly at a loss.

"You too." I grip my car keys tight in my hand and shift on my feet.

A wave of sadness drifts over me. I hate to admit it, but I'll miss seeing Ethan every day. I'd grown used to sharing that small space with him. We'd developed our own rituals and routines within those walls. Every morning when we'd leave for work, I'd duck under his arm as he held the front door open. Every evening, he'd turn on the bathroom light, a nightlight for me, before going to bed.

Over this last month, Ethan has protected me from loneliness. And during those nights that I slept next to him, the ones we never speak of, he's protected me from the sharp teeth of my nightmares.

This reminds me of another time Ethan protected me. Something I've been wanting to ask about for a long time. "You know when you were interviewing?"

He blinks, confused at my sudden change of topic. "Yeah. I remember everything about that day."

"I've been meaning to ask you about Patrick. Melanie said he called me an ice queen, and you defended me. Why'd you do that? I can take care of myself."

Stepping closer, invading my personal space, Ethan looks serious. His voice drops low and husky. "I know you can, Tiffy. You're a savage when you want to be. You're mistaken. I wasn't defending you. I was merely correcting Patrick."

He picks up a single lock of hair from my shoulder. It blazes scarlet in the late morning light. Running it through his fingers, Ethan bends his head so I'm staring straight into his smoky eyes.

He says softly, "You're no ice queen. You're pure fire."

With that, he drops my hair and leans in close, bringing his face right up to mine. His breath ghosts over my mouth. His amber eyes are all I can see. My lungs, my heart, my entire body freezes as his lips hover over mine. *Is he going to kiss me? Is this really happening?*

At the last possible second, he veers to the side and places a feather-light kiss on my cheek. Then he stands and walks away, calling over his shoulder as he goes, "See you back in Columbus. Drive safely in that death trap you call a car."

He leaves me there in the parking lot.

Speechless.

33

On the drive home, I think about the text messages I've been receiving. They must be from either Rafe or Shelly. But which one? And why? Are they warning me? Or threatening me? Either way, I can't let whoever it is interfere with my current life. My fists curl as I think about how hard I've worked to gain some security. Finally, I have a good job. I live in a safe place. For so long, those were my only goals.

But now, after living with Ethan, it occurs to me there are other things to wish for. Companionship, friendship, and maybe, someday…love? When I mentally replay the past month, reviewing and analyzing our conversations, it's easy to recall the husky warmth of Ethan's laugh, the sensation of my head on his shoulder, the weight of his muscular arm over my body.

Like living with you too, Sleeping Beauty, vanilla creamer, pure fire. What does it all mean? Is it possible Ethan likes me? Maybe even has romantic feelings for me? The way he pressed that kiss to my cheek. I can still feel the sensation of his lips, a phantom caress that lingers like silk on my skin. And what about the way he held me at night? As if I were something precious. Or was he playing with me? Trapped in an apartment for four weeks with no better way to amuse himself?

My mind goes back and forth, speculating.

The inevitable next question is, what do I feel for him? I evaluate how my body responded to his touch, the want and longing. For years, I've kept everyone away. Avoided entanglement, never trusting another person enough to risk getting hurt. With Ethan, I felt safe and comfortable. I think of us laughing together over some movie I forced him to watch. The way his eyes danced and how charming his lopsided smile was.

Mr. Chen used to talk about his dead wife with such respect and love that it made my heart ache. Certainly, there had to be men like Mr. Chen who could be trusted. Was Ethan one of them?

By the time I arrive home, I'm convinced that a future with Ethan is a possibility. One worth pursuing. I'll wait and see how he is now that we are back in Columbus, but I'm hopeful for the first time in a long time.

Ethan doesn't contact me.

Not that Saturday or Sunday. That's okay. It's the weekend, I reassure myself. He's probably tired after working so hard in Cleveland.

He doesn't call on Monday or Tuesday. That's okay. He's working at one of our other hospitals across town all week, so I didn't expect to see him.

When I still haven't heard from him by Wednesday, I'm so angry I want to set the world ablaze. Ethan said I was pure fire. Well, I'll show him that he was right.

He finally calls on Thursday. Twice. I don't pick up.

Not going to give him the satisfaction of a response. The silent treatment might be juvenile, but I don't care.

On Friday, Ethan sends a text.

Tiffy, everything OK?

No way am I going to tell him. How embarrassing would that be? *I thought for a second you liked me and I liked you back, but then I realized I'm a fool.* What am I? In middle school? No, thank you. Better to cut off this friendship or whatever it was now. That way, there can be no more confusion.

No more hurt feelings.

SINDERELLA

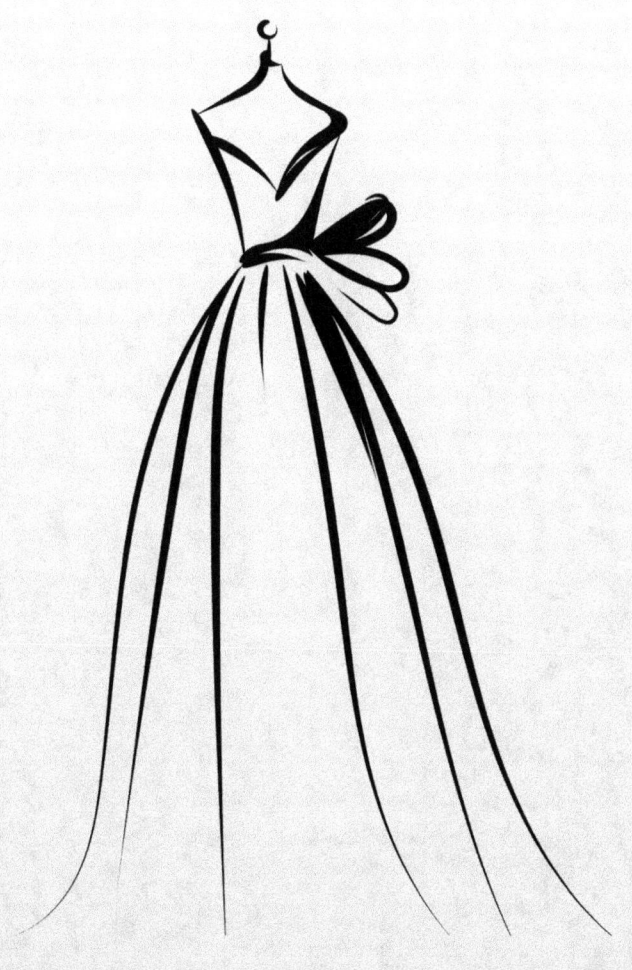

34

PAST, LAS VEGAS, NEVADA, AGE 16

Sixteen is not sweet for Shelly or me. In fact, it's the year that both of our lives fall apart.

That winter, Mike leaves Brandi.

The day after Mike and Brandi separate, Shelly and I sit at the ugly green tables in the center of our school. The tables are perforated, a multitude of tiny holes dotting their surface. Shelly has picked up a dry leaf. She shreds it into pieces and feeds it through the holes to watch the fragments drift to the ground.

"What happened with Mike?" I prod her.

She shakes her head mournfully. "He left because of me."

Images of Mike harassing Shelly are quickly discarded. Even though my mom had worried about it, I had never gotten the impression that Mike viewed us girls as sexual objects. I can't picture him hitting on Shelly.

She can see what I'm thinking. "No. Not like that. He told my mom he couldn't stand being tied down anymore. He wanted to explore the country. Mike said he still had feelings for her, but he was rotting away at our place."

Tiny pieces of leaf fall like rain through the holes. We watch them tumble down. Tears follow and hit the table with a metallic plop-plop. Shelly is crying silently.

"Mom blames me. It's not like she was crazy about me before this, but now every time she looks at me she sees the person who ruined her marriage. If she didn't have me, she would have followed Mike. They could have traveled the country together. She would have loved that. Once again, I've managed to destroy her life with my very existence. Since he left, all she does is lie around drinking and smoking pot. It's depressing."

I gently hug my friend, not sure how else to comfort her. Shelly buries her face in my neck to hide her sobs.

My world unravels in slow motion.

It begins with a cough. Then my mom lets out another cough and another. "It's just a bad cold. I'll be fine." Soon my mom is hacking so hard that it makes her feel faint. "I choked on something. Don't worry, Kitten."

She gets short of breath from walking up the stairs to our apartment. "Gotta exercise more. Mom's getting out of shape." She falls asleep on the couch every night, too tired to go to bed. "It was a long day at work."

When the Kleenex turns crimson from the blood she coughs up, we finally go see the doctor.

"I'm sorry," the doctor says. It's lung cancer. The less common and more aggressive kind. Small cell lung cancer. After a battery of tests, we find it's already spread. Tiny metastatic spots appear in her lymph nodes and bones. Like the tumors are alien space invaders intent on colonizing my mother's body.

The doctors ask my mom repeatedly, "Did you smoke?"

"Never," answers Mom.

The doctors look suspicious, like she must be lying.

"Could it have been the secondhand smoke from the casinos?" I ask.

The doctors shrug. "Could be. We won't ever know for sure."

The treatments start. Chemotherapy. Radiation.

The next year I spend in hospitals, surrounded by vases of red roses and cheerfully colored cards that say, "Get Well Soon." Mom won't ever get well. I know that. The constant beeping of the monitors still echoes in my ears on the rare nights I sleep at home alone or at Mr. Chen's. I become adept at doing my homework in the cafeteria or in my mom's room, sitting in uncomfortable plastic chairs. I miss so many days of school that the attendance officer automatically marks me as absent unless she hears otherwise.

With Mr. Chen's help, I learn about the labs and tests the doctors order for my mother. I know to ask about hemoglobin and hematocrit, to see how my mom's body is responding to blood loss.

The seeds of a desire to practice medicine that were planted deep in my subconscious with Mr. Chen's anatomy book now start to grow roots. I witness firsthand how important a doctor's job is, how a good doctor can spark hope even in the darkest times.

35

PAST, LAS VEGAS, NEVADA, AGE 17

On a rare day when I'm at school, I walk across the quad, glancing over my shoulder. I get this weird feeling sometimes, like I'm being watched. It must be paranoia, though. I don't see anyone staring at me. Shelly's sitting at our usual lunch table. It's a relief to see her familiar face, although, as I rush over to join my friend, I notice that she looks different. It's like she's aged in the time that we've been apart.

Shelly's dyed her hair beach blonde with chunky orange streaks. Her dark roots are a skunk's stripe close to her scalp. Thick black eyeliner and mascara emphasize her large brown eyes and the shadows beneath. A tight black ribbon acts as a choker necklace. Fishnet stockings rise out of black Doc Martens boots.

"Hey." I drop into the seat next to her. "I haven't seen you in forever. How's it going?" I've been so busy dealing with my mom's illness and trying to stay caught up at school that I'm losing touch with Shelly.

"Awful." There's a resigned hopelessness in her voice. "How about you?"

"Same."

"I think we might get evicted. There's no money left."

"I'm worried about that, too," I sympathize. "Our apartment manager is patient, but she won't wait forever if I can't make the rent." It gives me no relief to realize that Shelly and I are dealing with the same problems. Moms that can't or won't work and unending debt. It's too much for a 17-year-old to handle.

"I need money," I admit.

She examines me carefully. "How serious are you about wanting to make money?"

"I'm dead serious. We can't move out of that apartment. My mom's not strong enough to look for a new place." Even the overcast sky seems lower today. It's claustrophobic. The weight of the clouds presses down on my head.

Shelly glances around, like she wants to make sure no one can hear. In a whispery voice, she says, "I've got an idea."

36

PRESENT, COLUMBUS, OHIO

Not talking to Ethan doesn't make me feel any better. I robotically move through my day, going through the motions. When I interact with the staff, I'm cool and remote. At lunch, I eat by myself rather than at the table where Melanie and a large group of residents sit. Back to my default ice queen status. Glumly, I imagine placing a crown of icicles and thorns on my head.

The only thing that makes the day bearable is knowing that tomorrow I'll leave this place. It's time to go to the big annual American College of Advanced Radiology conference in Orlando, Florida. This year, the conference organizers have requested *me* as a guest speaker. It's rare for a resident to be asked to give a lecture, so I remind myself to double check that the renal tumor staging is accurate this time. I can't make a mistake. No Ethan will be around to correct...or embarrass me.

The best part about the conference is that it includes free Disney theme park tickets. Lectures end every day at 3:00 p.m., leaving plenty of time to check out the parks in the evening. Ever since I was a child watching cartoon movies and snuggling on the couch with my mom, I've dreamed of going to Disney World. Before, I couldn't afford it, but now I can go because the Medical Education Department pays for the conference entrance fees.

All I need to pay for is the airfare and hotel. I lucked out and found a cheap

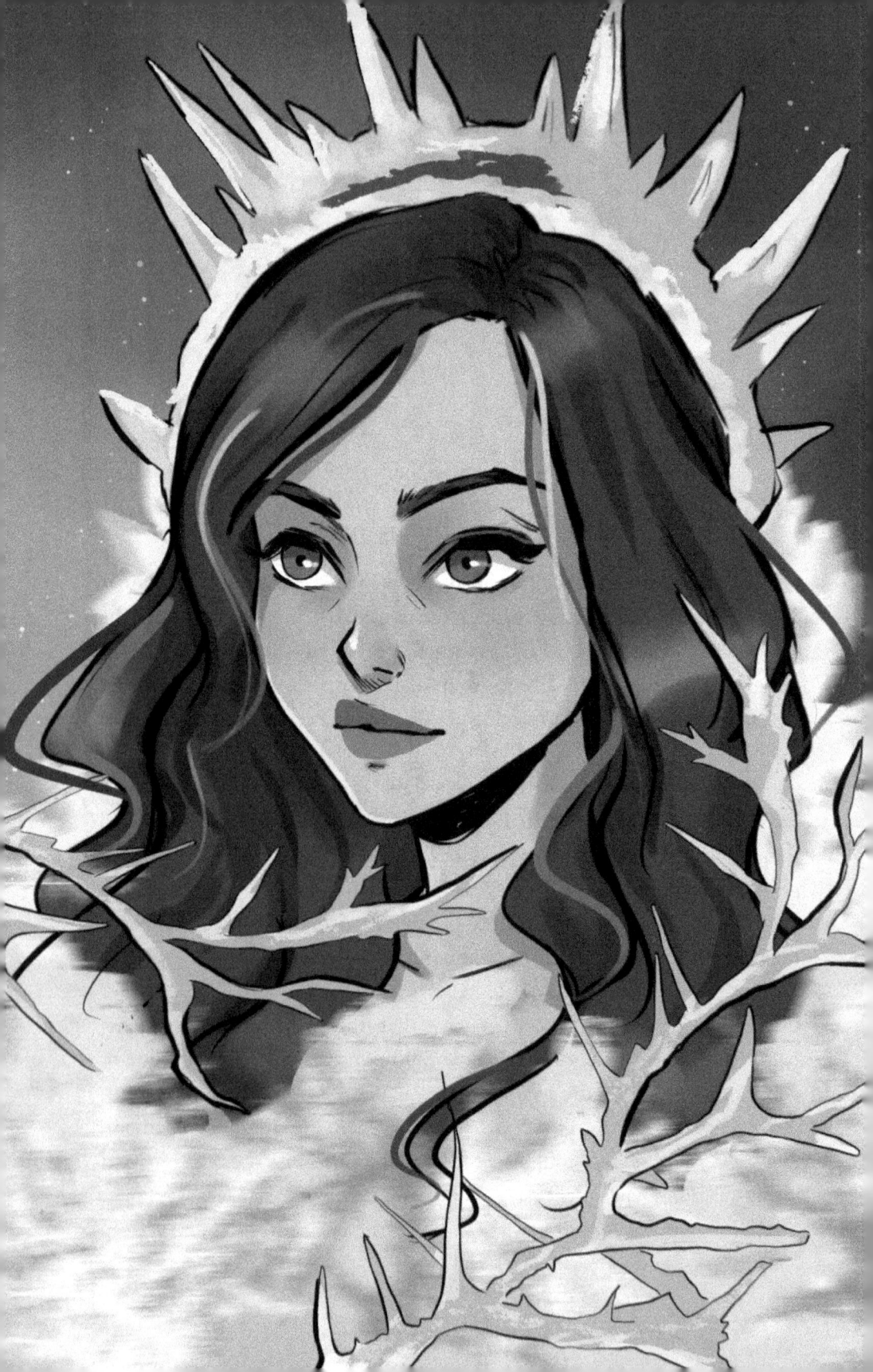

flight. The hotel room was a splurge, even with the discounted conference room rate, but it was worth it because it saved me from having to rent a car. It's the hotel where the conference is being held and has hourly buses leaving to take guests to the parks. I had hoped I would get the Resident of the Month award with its $1,000 bonus, but they haven't announced the winner yet. I'll have to pinch pennies and cover the cost on my own.

The timing couldn't be more perfect. Now I won't have to worry about seeing Ethan for an entire week.

* * *

"Flight 1312, please prepare for boarding." The airline agent's voice crackles through the speaker directly above my head. I sigh with relief. My flight is on time. I shouldn't worry since my presentation isn't until the middle of the week, but I don't want to miss a single day in the amusement parks.

The straps of my backpack dig into my shoulders as I board the plane. I shift it, adjusting the heavy bag. It's weighed down by my laptop and several romance books. The flight is packed. Angry babies wail as I walk by, their tight-lipped parents trying desperately to calm them. When I finally locate my seat, I'm disappointed to find it's on the aisle. Longingly, I gaze at the empty window seat. I hoped to sit there so I could watch take-off and landing.

I've only been on an airplane once before, when I moved from Las Vegas to Ohio. I still remember when the plane broke through the clouds. The way those gauzy wisps tore apart and then recoalesced. Too bad the human heart can't be punctured and then repatched so easily.

A thin man in a shabby black suit sits in the middle. I offer him my most friendly smile as I settle in next to him. He doesn't return the gesture. In fact, the man scowls at me.

Geez, Middle Man. What's your problem?

Ignoring him, I bring out my latest romance book. I've been looking forward to a couple of hours of uninterrupted reading. Hopefully, focusing on other people's love lives will keep my mind off Ethan.

When I've read about five pages, a body jostles against my legs as the passenger with the window seat attempts to climb over me. A heavy foot stomps on my toes. I let out a yip of pain, looking up angrily to see warm amber eyes staring down at me.

"I'm sorry," says Ethan. "Did I step on you?"

My mouth gapes open.

What the heck?

Ethan takes his place by the window. His ridiculously long legs don't fit the tight space, so his knees end up jammed against the seatback in front of him. It doesn't look comfortable, but I refuse to feel sympathy for him.

I lean forward, bending around Middle Man, and hiss loudly, "What are you doing here?"

Middle Man's head snaps toward me as he frowns with confusion and disapproval. "Do you two know each other?"

I say "no" at the same time that Ethan says "yes," which only deepens Middle Man's consternation.

"Well? Why are you here?" I demand again.

A subdued but calm Ethan leans forward, peering around Middle Man so he can meet my eyes. He whispers back, "I called Washburn yesterday and asked if I could go to the conference, told him I needed the continuing medical education credits. I wasn't sure if he'd say yes with such short notice."

A million questions run through my mind. "When did you get here? I didn't see you at the gate."

"I just found out that Washburn approved my request. By the time I packed and drove here, I was running late. I had to sprint through the entire airport. They closed the gate right behind me." Ethan wipes away a fine sheen of sweat from his brow.

The dream of a peaceful and relaxing flight evaporates in front of me. Now that the shock at seeing Ethan is wearing off, my anger comes raging back.

I glare at him. "Are you paying Dr. Washburn or something? How do I keep getting stuck with you?"

My voice rises higher in volume, earning a dirty look from Middle Man.

"I'm not paying him, but I probably should be." Ethan returns my look. "Anyway, I told you several times already that you're stuck with me."

"What does that even mean?" I clench my jaw in frustration.

Middle Man listens to our conversation with a sour expression. His annoyed stare shifts from my face to Ethan's. The fasten seat belt light dings overhead and illuminates.

Evading my question, Ethan narrows his eyes at me. "How about you tell me why you're mad at me. Let's start with that."

"I'm not mad at you. That would imply that I care, which I *don't*."

The plane taxis down the runway. Middle Man bends forward to open his bag at his feet. He blocks my view of Ethan, so I lean back to see around him. Ethan moves back as well and says, "Liar, you care so much that your face is turning the same shade as your hair. Talk to me. Tell me what I did wrong."

I take a sharp intake of breath, seething. "Don't you call me a liar." I'm gripping the metal armrest, my knuckles white. I'm so angry. My blood is boiling with it. "Ugh! I want to punch your stupid, handsome face right now."

"Punch away. It won't stop me from looking at you." Ethan sets his jaw, determination flaring in his amber eyes. Then that expression shifts into a small, satisfied smirk. He adds, "You just admitted I'm handsome."

Gah! He's infuriating! *Don't let him distract you with those pretty eyes and even prettier words*, I remind myself. Another set of eyes, another pretty mouth full of lies, had fooled me in the past.

Middle Man clears his throat loudly as if to remind us he's still there. At the front of the plane, the airline attendants demonstrate how to use a seat belt. "Hey. Do you mind?" Middle Man addresses me. "If you two need to talk, I can switch with you."

"No, thanks," I sniff. "No need to change seats." Still holding on to my fury, I glare at Ethan while answering Middle Man's question. "Besides, that man is the *last* person I want to sit with."

Ethan brushes aside my insult. He's relentless, wanting me to explain myself. "It's because I didn't call, isn't it?"

"How about you?" Middle Man asks Ethan. "Do you want to switch?" Ethan doesn't even glance in his direction. His eyes are only for me.

I can't hold back any longer. The memory of checking my phone every ten minutes to see if he'd called, of sleeping with it on the pillow next to my head, all comes rushing back. "Yes! I'm mad you didn't call. It was five days,

Ethan. Five days!" I want to scream at him, to rage, but I can't with all these people around. My hands ball into tight fists.

Ethan blows out an anguished breath and runs his hands through his hair. "I knew it was a lot up in Cleveland. I thought you might need some time alone, some space. The last thing I want is to overwhelm you and make you run, Tiffy."

Middle Man twists in his seat, looking like he'd rather be anywhere else. The pilot's voice comes through the loudspeaker and instructs the airline attendants to prepare for departure.

"Stop it. That's not my name," I snap.

Ethan continues as if he didn't hear me. "Has it occurred to you that maybe, just maybe, I hoped *you* would call *me?* Maybe you aren't the only one who's scared, the only one with something to lose." His hand comes up to rub the small scar in his eyebrow.

I see it then, a crack in his easygoing, charming exterior. I see Ethan's insecurity. His fear of failure. The puzzle pieces slide into place. He thinks he failed his family by not living up to their expectations. That he failed his teammates when he got hurt and quit baseball. That he failed the staff at Highview Hospital when he changed residencies and moved to Columbus.

For whatever reason, he's making an effort to be closer to me, and he's frightened of failing at that, too. I'm still mad that he didn't call, but now I understand it better. After all, I didn't call him either. I was too busy being a coward.

A well of sadness rises in me. I hate this. Hate fighting with him. I'm so tired of being angry, wary, and frightened. Tired of looking over my shoulder. It's exhausting. The only time I didn't feel that way was when I was with Ethan. I need that relief again, the calm he provides.

"You know what? There's an empty seat in that row over there. I'm going to go." Disgruntled, Middle Man gathers his things together. He stumbles over my foot as he leaves. That's the second time someone has stepped on my foot in less than ten minutes. I'm not sure which hurts worse, my toes or my heart.

Ethan moves into the newly vacated middle seat. In a softer voice, he says, "I'm sorry. I should have called sooner. Sometimes I overthink things. Make it more complicated than it needs to be. I didn't mean to upset you."

The plane picks up speed, its nose rising in the air as we lift off. The force presses Ethan and me into the cushions. Ethan's apologetic, open-palmed hand moves slowly toward me. I watch his advancing hand suspiciously, like it's a venomous snake, ready to strike and bite. He settles on top of my clenched fist. His fingers intertwine themselves into mine, pushing my fingers apart one by one until my hand relaxes.

It's like a miracle, his hand holding mine.

"You know why I asked to come to the conference?" Ethan's staring at me intently, his gaze searching my face.

I think I know the answer, but I'm too scared to say it.

What if I'm wrong?

"Why?" I ask instead.

"*You*. I'm here for *you*. I followed *you*." His fingers tighten around mine. More softly, he says, "I can't keep my eyes off *you*. That's why I'm here. I want a chance, Tiffy. Give it to me." Staring at me with those light liquid eyes, he pleads, he demands.

Unblinking, I stare back because, if I'm really being honest with myself, I can't take my eyes off him either.

We stay like that, our gaze and hands locked together for a long minute, until he says, "Let's call a truce. I don't want to fight."

A heavy band releases its grip from my chest. A long breath escapes me and, with it, the anger I've been holding onto this past week. "Okay." I'm distracted by Ethan's warm, rough palm lying nestled against mine.

The lopsided grin is back. An old friend I haven't seen since we left Cleveland.

Still calming myself, I deliberately slow my pulse and focus on him. He's making an effort. I recognize that now, and he deserves the chance he's asking for. "This is your first time at Disney World too?" I ask.

His face is so close I can see how his scar is puckered from where he had stitches. "Yeah. You know what I'm most excited about?"

"What?"

"Seeing it with you." He rubs his thumb lightly over the back of my hand, stirring butterflies in my stomach that flutter their wings and rise into my chest. "Will you go with me? To the parks?"

I hesitate. I'm not angry at him anymore, but I have a lot of unanswered questions. It's like we're circling around something big, something unnamed. I'm not blind to my growing attraction to Ethan. I'm swimming deeper into the ocean of my feelings and can no longer touch the sandy floor beneath my feet.

I pause, thinking. "Okay. On one condition."

"Which is?"

"We trade seats. I want the window."

The corners of his mouth rise higher into a sunny crooked smile. "Done."

It's true that I want the window seat, but the real reason I agree to go to Disney World with Ethan is simple. He's holding my hand, and it feels like a promise of something more. I want to find out what that something is.

I'm not running anymore.

37

PAST, LAS VEGAS, NEVADA, AGE 17

A few days later, I tell Mr. Chen I'm going to the library and ask him to keep an eye on my mom, who's asleep upstairs. But I don't go to the library. Instead, I walk to the parking lot, where Shelly is waiting in a beat-up sports car. I hop in, and we speed off.

Pulling my costume out of a plastic grocery bag, I shake it out, letting the glitter sparkle. Shelly and I went to a thrift store yesterday. With her help, I picked out a plain white bikini and knee-high white boots. Our next stop had been a craft store where we bought the fake diamond sequins, glitter glue, and large feathers that now adorn our outfits.

It had been fun. Shopping together. It'd been so long since I felt young, like a normal teenager. Being with Shelly, as we tried on every crazy outfit we saw, had made me giggle. It had been a tiny burst of freedom, away from the hospital and sickness. It reminded me that there was an entire world out there. One that didn't run on alarms set to give the next dose of medicine. A world where a girl can be carefree, for just a moment, and go shopping with her best friend.

I change as we zoom down the road, heading for the Strip. Shelly is already dressed, her feathered headband brushing against the roof of the car. Her outfit is all red. Red bikini top and bottom. Knee-high red boots so shiny they reflect the passing streetlights.

We're dressed like show girls. The kind that you see in those cheesy Las Vegas shows. With tall headbands and skimpy clothing.

I'm in white, like an angel.

Shelly is in red, like the devil.

That had been Shelly's idea. "It's perfect," she had told me as we searched through the racks of clothing at Goodwill. "Tourists come to Vegas to escape their boring lives. When they're here, it's like there's a devil on one shoulder telling them to do all the bad things, drink, gamble, cheat. On the other shoulder, there's an angel telling them to be good and resist temptation. That's us, the angel and the devil."

Once I'm dressed, I crack the car window open a bit. My cheeks are warm, and the cool breeze helps calm them. I bounce in my seat, a mixture of giddiness and trepidation warring within me. I feel guilty for lying to my mom and Mr. Chen. But there's also a sense of adventure, like the anticipation you get right before a school field trip. When you are with your friends, about to discover something new together.

"Tell me again exactly how this works," I ask, as the wind picks up empty candy wrappers at my feet and throws them up in the air like confetti. The wrappers swirl, caught in invisible vortexes, before falling back down.

Shelly checks the rearview mirror, then answers, "The tourists pay good money, cash, to take a picture with us. We stand on the Strip and wait for the vacationers. Those people want something to show what an amazing time they had here. They'll take that picture home and show it off. Let their friends see how great they look with two hot girls hanging off them. It's a souvenir *and* an ego boost."

"You sure we can make money? Like real money?" I ask, thinking about the growing pile of medical bills at home. The creditors have started calling, hounding me.

"Definitely." Shelly's confidence reassures me. Thank goodness we're doing this together. I wouldn't have been brave enough to come on my own.

Watching the candy wrappers dance, I ask, "Where'd you get this car, anyway? Is it new?" I've never seen her drive before. Brandi has one car, an old minivan, that she never lets Shelly use.

Shelly keeps her eyes on the road. "It's not mine. Just borrowed it from a friend."

"Oh, okay." I adjust the zipper on my boot, locking my foot more firmly in place. "Where are we going to park?"

"I'll leave our car over in the parking lot by the Starlight. I know how to get past the chain-link fence. We can walk up the Strip until we find a good area to attract tourists. It's too bad we're starting in the evening. Most of the good spots will already be taken. Some ladies who dress up as show girls are territorial," she explains.

We drive up to the Starlight, a casino and hotel complex on the northern end of the Las Vegas Strip that was built in the 1950s. A tall sign with its iconic star logo towers in front of the main entrance. The sign was once lit with many brightly colored bulbs but is now darkened forever.

The Starlight was abandoned years ago and has fallen into disrepair. When I've driven past it before, I've shivered, noticing the haunted feeling it gives off, like its guests past and present have left their mark. I imagine all the people who have laughed inside those walls and all the ones who have cried. The brides who got married in its wedding chapel and the men bankrupted at its gambling tables. How many people had their hearts broken in there?

Now the Starlight's guests consist of the homeless and underage teenagers looking for a place to party. When we get closer, I can see debris and graffiti along the edges of the building. Amorphous people-like shapes move in its shadows. Through my open window, I hear music so faint I can't make out the tune. The notes drift out from the structure and fade into the night.

It's eerie.

Shelly parks the car, and we walk across the street, then up the Strip. We go past the Tropicana, MGM, and Paris. Women and girls dressed like us are on every street corner. Finally, in front of Bally's Hotel, there's an empty section of sidewalk.

Now that I'm out in public wearing my scanty costume, my nerves kick in. I've never felt more exposed. The warm Vegas breeze crawls around me, tickling every inch of bare flesh. It's hard to resist the urge to cross my arms across my overly accentuated cleavage. The boots are already pinching my heels. I have that sense again, of being watched, but that's not surprising, given what I'm wearing.

It doesn't take long to get our first customers. A group of five college-age men approach. Shelly shrewdly evaluates them as they come closer. I hang back, letting her make the sale. I'm impressed when she tells them it'll be $10 each to take pictures. Fifty dollars is a lot of money, so I brace for them to reject the offer. Instead, the men dig around in their pockets and hand over $50 of crumpled bills without hesitation.

They have regular cameras and a Polaroid. The men ask a random passerby to stop and take the pictures. After some scrambling, they arrange themselves in an uneven line, with Shelly and me as bookends. Arms are thrown over each other's shoulders, and everyone smiles.

"Cheese," says the man next to me, with whiskey on his breath. Click, click, click. Camera flashes go off one after another, blinding me. We do a few different poses, rearranging ourselves between each shot. After we're done taking pictures, we gather with the group of men to look at the Polaroid images. Our faces slowly come into focus, like ghosts materializing into existence.

I almost don't recognize myself. I hadn't realized how much I've grown over the past year. In my tight bikini, I can see how my legs are now long and tapered and my hips and bust have filled out into soft curves. The push-up top mounds my breasts together until they create a deep valley of cleavage.

I look hot.

The guys offer Shelly one of the Polaroid photos, which she accepts. With good-bye waves and a chorus of "thank you," the men leave.

"That wasn't so bad, was it?" Shelly asks before turning to greet the next group. This time it's a couple of gray-haired men. Nice grandfatherly types in town for a conference who tip an extra $10.

We're a hit. A steady stream of people want to get their picture taken with us. It's mostly men, although the occasional bachelorette or woman's birthday party comes along. My cheeks ache from all the fake smiling. Shelly and I have just stopped for the night when a deep voice asks harshly behind me, "What's *she* doing here?"

I pivot to see Rafe standing a foot away. He's glowering at me. Last week at school his hair was overgrown and shaggy, but now it's been buzz cut, his scalp shining through. I want to run my hand over it to see if the short hairs will feel prickly on my palm like I suspect. I've watched him from afar for so long that being close to him now is surreal.

Rafe turns his glare to Shelly and repeats, "Why is she here?"

His anger at my presence makes me defensive. Does he hate me? Maybe he resents or, even worse, regrets saving me?

Shelly bristles at his tone. She spits back, "Tiffany's here because I asked her to come. The tourists expect to take pictures with two girls. Not one. We've made almost $1,000 tonight." She discreetly pulls the wad of cash out of her purse and flashes it at Rafe as proof.

Rafe just grunts when he sees the money. "It's a bad idea. She doesn't belong."

His attitude is getting under my skin, so I speak up. "The 'she' you keep referring to is standing right here. I can go anywhere I like. Last time I checked, this is a free country."

Green eyes shift to pierce me. "This is what you want?" he demands. "To be out here letting strangers grope you?"

"No one's groped me tonight." Except for a drunk bachelor, but I keep that to myself. "Even if they did, I can handle it," I add with more bravado than I feel.

A disbelieving laugh from Rafe. "Yeah. Right." His eyes move up and down my body, evaluating me, but not in a sexy way like the other men from this evening. He looks at me like he's looking for weakness, for my flaws. Whatever he sees must displease him because he frowns and turns away, dismissing me.

"It's late. You should go," Rafe gruffly tells Shelly.

"We were just packing it in anyway. Come on, Tiffany." Shelly throws her backpack over one shoulder and tucks her jacket under her arm.

We walk silently to her car. Rafe follows us from a distance. He watches until we get safely into our seats and lock the doors. Then he disappears, dissolving into the shadows.

Back at my apartment, Shelly gives me half of the money. It's almost $500, mostly in $10s and $20s. I clutch the thick stack of bills tightly in my hand, the paper crinkling from my grip, and sigh in relief.

38

We put on our angel and devil show-girl outfits and go down to the Strip as often as we can. The money and the flexibility of going whenever we want are too good to stop. Soon, we stake out our own block just outside of the New York–New York hotel and casino. A miniature Lady Liberty casts her shadow over us as we work, making the perfect backdrop for tourists eager to snap a picture. The happy screams of roller-coaster riders echo over our heads.

I jokingly refer to this slice of sidewalk as our "office." At school, I'll ask Shelly if we are going into the "office" that night. It's a secret word between us, a code we can use without announcing our intentions to anyone else.

It's been nice to reconnect with Shelly. We're spending so many nights together that it's like the clock hands have moved backward. Back to the time when we were sisters in every way except by blood.

Rafe makes frequent appearances on the Strip. Sometimes I spot him far down the street, talking to people or lounging around. He's different every time I see him, changing his hair and clothing the way a snake sheds its skin. I admire that about him, how he doesn't cling to tradition or routine.

I'm not like that. I get nervous when my mom cuts my hair at our scarred kitchen table. "Just a little trim, Mama. Not too much."

Often, Rafe wanders down to us. He talks about school or makes sarcastic comments about the tourists who walk by. Rafe and Shelly have mutual friends, kids from Shelly's apartment complex that she moved into after her mom got married. People I don't know. Sometimes they talk about these friends. It makes me feel left out, how they have things in common I can never be a part of.

Quite a few kids from my high school haunt the Strip like street waifs from a Dickens novel. Some are there to kill time, some to buy drugs, and some to sell them.

I get further proof that Rafe is selling drugs. He does a lot of extended handshakes paired with meaningful eye contact. It's awfully suspicious. When he's down at our end of the Strip, he glowers at the men who come to take pictures with us. Eventually, Shelly demands he leave and stop scaring our customers away.

• • •

One Friday night, Shelly and I are walking back to the car when we see Rafe heading in the same direction. Shelly calls out his name.

The air has grown chilly. Shelly and I wear oversized jackets to keep warm and hide our skimpy bikinis. The feathers and gaudier parts of our costumes are put away in backpacks that bounce against our backs as we walk. Clutching our jackets tighter, we quicken our pace.

Rafe silently waits for us to catch up.

"Where're you going?" asks Shelly.

I'm still uncertain around Rafe, so I stay quiet.

"The Starlight. They're having a party." He gives us an appraising look and hesitates. "Do you want to come? A ton of people will be there."

"I don't think—" Shelly begins to say, but I cut her off.

"We can go." I ignore the shock on Shelly's face. She's always asking if I want to get food or ice cream on the way home from the Strip. I tell her no, citing reasons like homework and wanting to be with my mom.

The difference between those times and this one is that *Rafe* is going to the party. I'm tired of watching him from a distance. I want to get a closer look, maybe spend some time with him. It bothers me that he doesn't like me, and I need to know why. In my fantasies, I still see myself breaking down his walls. Like he has built himself a fortress, and I will be the sledgehammer to smash it into pieces.

Shelly's been dyeing her hair different colors. Today it's a purple-blue. Twirling her midnight-colored hair on a finger, she regards me with suspicion. "Are you sure, Tiffany? Don't you have a biology test on Monday?"

I do have a test on Monday. A big one. But how often am I going to have this opportunity? I'm tired of always being so responsible, of putting my mom and my academics first. The kids at that party aren't worrying about getting into college. They're out having fun and living in the moment.

For this one night, I want to be like them.

Playing it cool, I say, "I have all weekend to study. Besides, we can just stay for a little while. Okay, Shelly?" She drove us here. She's the one I need to convince.

"I'm fine with staying if you are." She shrugs, still looking at me like she knows I'm up to something but can't quite figure it out.

Even though he invited us, Rafe hesitates, giving me one last reluctant glance before we step into the Starlight. I've never been inside the dilapidated building before. The scene looks like something out of a horror movie. Debris and trash litter the floor. Graffiti climbs across the closed elevator doors. Faded and torn sunset red wallpaper hangs in long strips, peeling off the walls. There must still be electricity to the hotel because a mismatched collection of floor lamps scattered around the lobby emits random pools of light. Not exactly a "party" type of atmosphere.

This gloomy ambiance doesn't stop the people gathered in clusters throughout the room. They drink, smoke, and laugh with abandon. Someone has set up a boombox in the corner. It pumps out heavy techno dance music with bass so loud it reverberates through the soles of my shoes.

As soon as we enter the party, Rafe disappears. Within minutes, he's back bearing a gift. He hands Shelly an unopened bottle of wine. I've never seen wine like this before. It's cotton candy pink. Shelly looks at the label and nods approvingly, like she's some fancy sommelier. Wasting no time, she unscrews the cap and takes a big swig straight from the bottle. Wiping her mouth with the back of her hand, she passes it over to me.

I hold the wine up to the sporadic light, turning it this way and that to read the label. *Boone's Strawberry Hill*. I've never had alcohol before, never wanted it, but I feel the weight of Shelly's and Rafe's stares, so I take a timid sip. It tastes sweet, like liquefied candy, with a sour fermented aftertaste.

"Not bad," I admit.

Laughing loudly, Shelly snatches the bottle out of my hands. "Not bad? Is that all you can say? This stuff is freaking delicious. It's as easy on your throat going down as it is when it's coming back up."

"Eww, Shelly. Gross." My lip curls in disgust.

She laughs and takes another gulp. The casual way that she's drinking makes me think she's no stranger to alcohol. It strikes me that Shelly has a life beyond me. One we don't talk about much. Full of friends and activities I know nothing about. What else does my best friend do when we're apart?

Shelly hands me back the bottle. Emboldened, I drink a mouthful and then another. The wine has an acidic sting going down my throat. I evaluate myself. Am I drunk yet? How long does it take to detect the effects of alcohol? So far, I feel the same as usual. It's almost disappointing.

Shelly waves to friends from her apartment building and goes over to them. Rafe leans against the wall next to me with his arms crossed over his chest, watching the crowd like a king surveying his kingdom. I rack my brain, trying to think of something witty to say, but come up blank. He makes me nervous, a tantalizing kind of anxious excitement. It's a feeling I hate and love at the same time.

Finally, he cuts the silence. "What are you doing here, Tiffany?" His eyes stay fixed on the crowd in front of us.

My first response is pure relief that he remembers my name. The last time he said it out loud was when he rescued me. My second thought is anger at his disdainful tone. It's like he's judging me. He barely knows me, so he has no right to make assumptions. I lean back against the wall next to him and cross my arms over my chest, hugging myself. "My mom got sick. Cancer. I need money to pay the bills."

Rafe lets out a low, harsh bark of laughter. "We all need money." A lazy wave of his hand to indicate the crowd. "That's why we're all here, isn't it?" His hand drops back down to his side like it's too heavy to keep holding up. "I just thought you'd find a better way to get it. A smarter way."

"What smarter way?" I rotate toward him, a moth drawn to his flame.

"I don't know. You're the brainiac. Not me." Rafe continues to study the people gathering in front of us. More teens have joined the party now. I've lost sight of Shelly. Too many people block my view. Someone turns the music up even louder. Kids dance frantically to the heavy beat.

"Why? You don't want me here?" Sadness tingles in the back of my throat. I'm certain he's rejecting me.

Brilliant green eyes shift over to mine. They glitter in the lamplight, feral and fierce. "You don't belong here. You belong somewhere better." He sounds so certain.

"What do you mean by better?" I clench my fists tight with frustration.

His eyes drill into me like he can convince me with the intensity of his gaze. "I mean *better*. Away from here. Away from us."

There it is. The opportunity I've been waiting for. "What if I don't want to be away from you?" Standing on the street in a bikini has given me a newfound sense of self-confidence. My developing body used to scare me, but now that I've made money taking pictures with strangers, I see that my body can be a tool, a weapon even, used to get what I want.

An unfamiliar boldness overcomes me. Maybe it's the alcohol in my veins or maybe it's a year of pent-up longing. Either way, I'm taking advantage of this moment. I'm done daydreaming. I push off the wall and move to stand in front of him. In slow motion, I let my jacket casually slip off one shoulder, leaving it bare. Rafe's razor-sharp eyes follow the motion. I watch with satisfaction as he licks his lips, a hungry look stirring to life. His eyes flick back to me and narrow. He knows I did it on purpose.

"You should stay away from me," he warns again.

"No." I know he's bad, but he does it so well I don't care. Playing with fire, I step closer, between his legs, trapping him between my body and the wall. A profound sense of power thrills through me as the pace of his breathing quickens. It confirms I'm not the only one feeling the pulse between us. I hold still, delicately balanced inches away from him.

Rough hands move too fast for me to follow, grabbing my upper arms and pulling me to him. Rafe kisses me, or maybe I kiss him. It's all too quick and overwhelming to figure out the details. All I know is his lips are on mine, his hard body crushing me as he holds me close. Calloused fingers move, burrowing into my hair as he deepens the kiss. He tastes sweet, some liquor I don't recognize.

My heartbeat thunders in my ears while Rafe's heart pounds under my hands. A fire that I haven't felt before ignites deep inside me. I've never felt so out of control, so not myself. His mouth is ravenous, sliding along my jaw to graze my earlobe. His lips continue their tour down my neck and then return to mine, bruising in their aggression. He's awakened something deep inside of me, something that makes me want this kiss to go on and on.

Loud voices raised in argument end the kiss all too soon. Shelly's voice, slurring. My head whips up and swivels until I find my friend arguing with a man. Shelly's face is flushed maroon, and her jaw is tight with anger. She stalks toward the man with her arm raised like she might strike him.

Rafe leaves me and marches across the room to retrieve an irate Shelly, dragging her back to where I wait. She sways on her feet, clearly drunk, the near-empty wine bottle dangling from her fingertips.

"Shelly? Why were you fighting with that guy?" I ask.

"He said my hair is ugly," Shelly yells, scowling, "that jerk."

"Okay. Calm down." I grab Shelly's arm and draw her close, restraining her.

Unflustered, Rafe tells me, "Come on. I'll drive you both home."

"What about Shelly's car? She drove here. I would take us, but it's a stick shift. I don't know how to drive it." Shelly sways drunkenly in my arms.

"I'll make sure her car gets home." He motions to a guy I didn't notice before. The man comes over, and Rafe whispers to him. Immediately, the stranger gets Shelly's keys out of her backpack and leaves. I watch the whole interaction with unease. How the man was so deferential toward Rafe unnerves me. It was like he was just standing around, waiting for Rafe's next command.

The three of us leave the party and walk through the crowded parking lot to Rafe's truck. Along the way, Shelly systematically tries to open the door handles of each car as we walk past. When the passenger door of a small red sports car pops open, she squeals with delight. She scrambles into the car and begins pawing through every seat and cupholder.

My mouth gapes with disbelief. "Shelly, what are you doing?"

Continuing her investigation of the glove compartment, she slurs. "Let's see what we can find." A drunken shout sounds out from the car as she pulls $5 out of the glove compartment. "Look at this!" She waves the bill in the air, grinning, then shoves it into her pocket.

I protest. "You can't do that."

Shelly's voice is muffled as she bends down to look under the car's seats. "If they're dumb enough to leave their car unlocked, then they're asking for this. Don't worry. I won't take anything too valuable. Once I saw a lady's diamond engagement ring sitting in a cupholder, and I just left it," she says as if that excuses the petty theft she's doing.

Wait. She's done this before?

I glance at Rafe to see his reaction, hoping he'll back me up and get her to stop this madness. But his face is impassive, and he slows to let Shelly do her work.

I try again to get her to stop.

"Don't be such a goody-two-shoes," she tells me. "No one's going to miss this stuff. You know I need it a lot more than they do."

Finding two more unlocked cars, she steals from each of them. My stomach has turned sour, either from the strawberry wine or watching my best friend rob strangers.

The car ride to my apartment is silent as a tomb. Shelly stares out the window, clutching her belly like she might hurl. Rafe's truck may not be fancy, but I still don't want it decorated with the Spaghetti-O's she and I ate before we left for the Strip.

At my parking lot, I help Shelly down. Leaning back into the cab, I say good-bye to Rafe and then pause. I want to say something poignant, given our epic kiss earlier, but insecurity keeps me silent. I wonder, does he regret it now?

The dim glow of the streetlights doesn't reach into the dark truck. Rafe is wreathed in shadows, his expression hidden. Just when I'm about to retreat, he reaches out and gently grazes the back of his knuckles along my cheek and down to my jawline. His voice is as rough as his hands. "Night, Tiffany."

"Good night," I whisper, breathless from his touch. A minute later, he's gone, his broken taillight flashing once before he pulls onto the main street. I stare after him, hand pressed to my cheek, which burns from his caress. My fingers move to my lips, bruised from my first kiss.

39

PRESENT, ORLANDO, FLORIDA

After checking into our hotel, Ethan and I decide to go to Magic Kingdom since it's the original Florida park. The bus is crowded, and the road is bumpy. We sit side-by-side, jostling into each other with every turn. After one particularly sharp corner, Ethan puts his arm around me, pulling me close. "For stability," he tells me. This bus full of crying babies and tired tourists should be the least romantic place on Earth, so why is my heart thrumming?

Dappled, shifting sunlight comes in through the bus windows. It plays across Ethan's face and adds auburn highlights to his hair. A few strands fall into his eye, and he sweeps them aside, tilting his head back. I stare, captivated by the shadow of his jaw, the movement of his throat as he swallows. My blood pulses when his fingers tighten on my hip with each swerve in the road. I'm almost sad when the bus ride is over and we're deposited at the large iron gates that lead into the park. As we walk through the turnstiles, my eyes widen.

There it is. Magic Kingdom.

Tourists wait in lines to take pictures by the iconic, gray-roofed train station. The tantalizing smell of fresh popcorn drifts through the air. Children happily shriek and dart between their parents' legs.

A parade passes by in front of us. Large floats full of beloved Disney characters go by while accompanying music pours out of speakers attached to filigreed lamp posts. The last float in the cavalcade has sorcerer Mickey Mouse waving to the crowd with his pointed wizard hat perched tall on his head. I wave back like I've seen a long-lost friend.

We've only been in the park for five minutes, and already I'm so happy. There's a certain magic in the air. The happiness of thousands of vacationers all jammed together spreads from one person to another until we are all bathed in it, this communal joy.

The parade finishes and heads away, the music fading from the loudspeakers. Beaming, I turn to find that Ethan is watching me rather than the parade. He has a bemused expression on his face, his lopsided smile gentle and his eyes warm.

"What?" I'm suddenly self-conscious under his gaze.

Ethan shakes his head slightly. "Nothing. It's just that I've never seen you look…"

"Look what?" I ask sharply.

"So happy," he says simply. "I've never seen you so carefree and happy."

"Oh." I don't quite know how to respond to his compliment.

Snapping his focus away from me, Ethan stands tall and surveys Main Street. He squares his shoulders. "Where should we start? We need a game plan."

I'm all business now. "Don't worry. I've memorized the park maps."

"Wait, you *memorized* them?" Ethan asks incredulously.

"Memorized," I confirm.

"Like all four parks? You memorized the maps for *all* of them?"

"Try to keep up, Ethan. Yes, I didn't want to waste time looking at a map. I want to optimize every minute we have." Looking around, I get my bearings. "We should move through the park clockwise, so we end up in Tomorrowland."

"Sounds good to me." Before Ethan can take a step in that direction, I halt him with my hand in the air.

"First, let me download the Disney app onto your phone. You can use my account so we can reserve rides and order food for each other. That way I can look up wait times for the rides on my phone while you reserve them on yours. It'll be more efficient."

I take Ethan's phone and type in my username and password. It's the same one I use on all my accounts—that way I never forget it. Once I have Ethan's app set up correctly, I hand the phone back.

"Ready to go?" I'm almost bouncing in my excitement.

"You lead, and I'll follow," says Ethan. "Just like in the hospital."

We smile at each other, remembering those early training days.

Before we go on any rides, we get a churro. It's warm and soft on the inside with a hint of outside crunch. Licking the sugar off my fingers, I stroll down Main Street. My head swivels, taking in every detail from the old-fashioned storefronts to the elaborate window displays. When the crowd clears enough that I can see the castle in the center of the park, I come to a standstill, staring. The castle is beautiful, with twirling towers of pink and blue. Ornate gold spires sit atop each tower, bearing flags that flap jauntily in the breeze.

It's almost too pretty to be real.

The image blurs as tears fill my eyes.

Ethan's by my side instantly. "Tiffy? What's wrong?"

I sniffle. "I'm sorry. My mom would have loved it here so much. She was the one who introduced me to Disney. She adored all those old stories of Princesses kissing their Prince Charmings. True love that lasts forever."

A tear slides down my cheek, and Ethan chases it with his fingertip. I tilt my head up to see him better and try to explain. "It's not that I'm sad to be here. I'm just sad to be here without *her*. Does that make any sense?"

He tugs me into his arms, lending me his warmth. I close my eyes and breathe in his clean, minty scent. I'm pressed against his chest, and his deep voice vibrates under my ear. "Of course it does. It's natural to miss her. I'm sure she would love to see you here, surrounded by characters that you watched together. I imagine your mom would be proud of you. How smart, strong, and successful you are."

I peer up at him, so tall and confident. I've wondered that before. If my mom would be proud of me. I think she would like my job because she always wanted me to care for others. But she would be disappointed in parts of my past. In the bad things I did, even though I did them for her. Ethan doesn't know about those times, so I can't correct him.

It's weighing on me. The closer we get, the more I will lose if Ethan finds out about me. What would he think if he knew about my times on the Strip? Would it sully my image? Would he reject me? It's too big of a risk. I can't tell him, but the longer I wait…if he finds out, the worse it will be.

I shake my head and pull out of his arms. These are not the things I want to think about during my first trip to Disney World. Dashing the last of my tears away, I say in an overly bright voice, "I'm fine. Let's go." I whirl around and take off down the street, with a concerned-looking Ethan following behind me.

Luckily, the sights of Magic Kingdom distract me from my sadness. Ethan and I go into Adventureland first, where we ride Pirates of the Caribbean and the Jungle Cruise. On the Jungle Cruise, the pilot of the boat cracks corny jokes. He says, "You know why a tiger has stripes, right? It's to avoid being spotted." Ethan snorts with laughter when he hears that and elbows me until I'm laughing along with him.

Next, we walk past Liberty Square and get in line to ride the Haunted Mansion. Ethan stares at the spooky manor surrounded by graveyards. "Kinda creepy, isn't it?"

Blinking in the bright sunlight, I look up at the Gothic brick building with its ornate tower and gables. "It is eerie, but I've seen places way scarier than that."

"Oh yeah, like where?" he challenges.

"When I was in high school, kids used to party at this big old abandoned hotel and casino on the Las Vegas Strip. It was called the Starlight." It feels strange to say the name out loud. *Starlight*. I haven't spoken that word in years. All those terrible memories from the abandoned hotel have held such sway over me, but maybe if I speak the name some of that power will leech away. Hopefully, the Starlight will stop being a boogie man in my mind and return to the dilapidated building it really is.

"Yeah?" Ethan cocks his head, intrigued.

I nod, suppressing a shudder. "It was spooky inside, with peeling wallpaper and spider webs. I always thought it would be the perfect location for a horror movie."

"You partied there when you were in high school? I hadn't pegged you as the wild drunk girl type." He quirks his eyebrow at me.

"Don't get too excited." I roll my eyes. "It was one time, and I didn't even finish my drink." I remember the sweet-sour strawberry wine, can almost taste it on my tongue.

"Ah man, I was thinking I would get some good blackmail stories about high-school Tiffany," he teases, bumping his shoulder gently into mine.

"Sorry to disappoint, but I was pretty boring in high school," I lie as images of my angel costume, Rafe's brooding green eyes, and faces wearing elegant masks flip through my mind, like photographs in an old picture book. I take those memories, shove them in a mental drawer, and slam it shut.

40

PAST, LAS VEGAS, NEVADA, AGE 17

For all the times I go to the Strip, there are an equal number of times that I don't. Times when my mom needs me or I have too much homework or a test to study for. I'm still trying to maintain good grades. It must be working because my guidance counselor at school feels confident that I'll get lots of college acceptances, even to the Ivy League schools. My applications are in. Now I'm just waiting to hear back.

"School's the most important thing, Kitten," Mom reminds me, even when she's in the hospital.

Shelly has given up any pretense of caring about school. I see the big red Fs on the tests that get returned to her in class. Those nights when I don't make it to the Strip, she still goes. We've spent so much time there that we've made friends with the casino staff. The blackjack dealers, restaurant hostesses, spa masseuses, and club bouncers. A barter system exists between these workers. Concert tickets are traded for seats at the latest hot restaurant. Working an extra shift on the casino floor might get you a free facial at the spa, if you know the right people.

I miss a week with Shelly when my mom goes to the hospital for a bout of pneumonia. Once Mom is feeling better, the need for money forces me into my angel show-girl costume. I call Shelly to tell her I'm ready to go back to work.

That night, Shelly picks me up in a sleek, brand-new Mercedes. Much like

Shelly's hair color, her cars are always changing. Green hair and blue sedan today. I'm not an idiot. I understand these cars are probably stolen. The thing I don't know is how deep Shelly's involvement goes. Is she part of an international auto theft ring? Or is she hot-wiring cars on her own? Is Rafe involved?

These are questions I think about but never ask out loud. There's a precarious balance between Shelly and me, one I don't want to break. Financially, I can't risk losing her as my business partner. Emotionally, I can't risk losing her as my only friend.

I also can't risk being involved. Not with my future at stake.

After I've settled into the springy passenger seat, I inhale a deep lungful of new car smell. Shelly shifts the car into gear, and I get a glimpse of a large black stamp in the shape of an RA on the back of her hand.

"What's that all about?" I ask, pointing to the letters. They remind me of a logo, but I can't remember which one.

A half-shrug from Shelly. "It's a club at the Luxor. I went last night."

"How'd you get in?" I grab her hand, forcing her to steer one-handed, and pull it close to my face, inspecting the blurred letters. "You don't have an ID."

The passing street lamps create a strobe pattern in the car's interior, throwing it into alternating periods of illumination and shadow as we pass in and out of pools of light.

"I do now." Her white teeth gleam as she breaks into a self-satisfied smile.

"What?" I drop her hand, and she places it back on the steering wheel. "How?"

The smile widens into a grin. "You remember the bouncer over at the Rio? Bruce?"

I nod, picturing the tattooed man in his slick black suit. "Yeah, I know him."

"He hooked me up." She glances toward the passenger seat. "He can get you a fake ID, too. I only paid $30."

"No, thanks." I shake my head. I've curled my hair tonight, so the movement sends my ruby-red spirals bouncing.

"Why not? I've been going to the clubs, and it's fun. If you get an ID, we can go together." Her voice becomes pleading. "Please?" she whines. "It'll be even better with you there."

"Sorry, but I can't. I'm trying to be there for my mom as much as possible." A twist of resentment stirs in my gut. Of course, I want to be out having fun too, but I have responsibilities. Of all people, I hoped Shelly would understand.

I freeze at her next words.

"Rafe was at the club last night, wearing this tight shirt. He must be working out because he's all bulked up. I'm telling you, he was looking good." She drags out the last word, practically salivating.

I still haven't mentioned my fascination with Rafe to Shelly. Something's been holding me back. I used to tell her everything, all my deepest, darkest secrets back when we were little kids, but not anymore. I flash back to the night she stole from cars in the Starlight parking lot. It made me uncomfortable to see that side of her, the lying and thieving side. Now it's too late to make a claim on Rafe. It's not like he belongs to me, anyway. We just shared one kiss.

"Oh?" I try to sound noncommittal, like I don't care, when in reality I'm hanging on every word she says. "He was there?"

"He was there looking hot," confirms Shelly with a Cheshire-cat grin. "I didn't get to talk to him, but next time I'll make sure he notices me."

A fiery knife twists in my heart. I turn to my window and open it halfway, using the motion to hide the tale-tell jealousy on my face.

Oblivious, she continues, "Guess who else was at the club?"

"Who?" Neon lights flash by outside my window. The sidewalks are crowded with tourists and revelers who stumble drunkenly down the street. It's noisy. As we drive past, music blares from restaurants and shops, each song overlapping with the next. The clinking sound of slot machines pours out of open casino doors. Every day is the same here, like it's an eternal Saturday night. The perfect night to go out and gamble with your money and sometimes with your heart, too.

"That guy who has a crush on you. You know the one. Short and geeky. What's his name again?" She turns the car into the Starlight parking lot, past the chain-link fence that's been cut and dragged away to leave an opening. Even though this lot is supposed to be blocked off, it's always full of cars. Nobody seems to care if we park here or that kids party in the abandoned hotel. I've never seen security around the place. There are rumors it's set for demolition. Supposedly, the plan is to implode the old hotel and casino using dynamite, but they haven't announced a date yet.

"Do you mean Stewart?" I answer Shelly's question.

I had met Stewart a few months ago. It had been late one night when the crowd was slow. Taking advantage of the lull, I had spread my jacket on the ground, sticky from spilled drinks, old gum, and who knew what else. I sat down and leaned against the cold concrete wall of the casino with my novel in hand when a voice interrupted me.

"Is that Harry Potter?"

I looked up to see a slim young man with black-rimmed glasses, which magnified his doe-brown eyes. He had wiry brown hair prematurely receding in the front. A sports jacket was thrown over a plaid button-up shirt paired with dark blue jeans and scuffed white sneakers.

"It's the third one." I held up *Harry Potter and the Prisoner of Azkaban* for the stranger to see.

"How do you like it? I've read them all, and this story is the darkest." Although he looked young, the man had a formal way of speaking, almost like a professor.

No one else I knew had read the series, so I was eager to discuss them. "I like it. I can't believe they executed the hippogriff, Buckbeak, though."

"Ah, keep reading. That part of the story isn't over yet." The man looked at the ground shyly. "I'm Stewart. I…I just graduated from college, and now I…I work at the Luxor." He had a slight stutter, like he wasn't sure what to say.

"Tiffany. I work…here I guess." I waved at the busy sidewalk in front of us.

Stewart's gaze followed my hand and then returned to me. "How do you like that? Working here?" he had asked hesitantly.

I searched his expression for judgment. I got that a lot from women who would wrinkle their noses like they smelled something rancid when they walked by me. People who looked down on me for my skimpy outfit and the fact that I was exchanging my looks for cold, hard cash. It used to bother me, that disdain on people's faces, but, over time, I had grown more comfortable with it. Whenever it became too much, I pictured my mom pale and fragile in a hospital bed, red hair blazing against the stark white pillow, and the money I needed to pay her medical bills. The image served as motivation to look past the revulsion.

No judgment was on Stewart's face, though. He seemed curious. Like my opinion was interesting and worthy of his attention. It had been a while since anyone had looked at me like that. We had talked for over an hour that night, mostly about books we liked and movies we'd seen. We quickly agreed that most movies made from books were disappointing. They could never compare to the pictures we had formed in our minds while reading.

I had seen Stewart a few times since then. He would seek me out, patiently waiting until there was a break in the stream of tourists shooting photos with me. I had an inkling he had a crush on me. He was an obviously intelligent guy, but his words would grow clumsy around me. The way his face would redden, and how he couldn't look me in the eye, were more clues.

I liked Stewart. He differed from most of the self-serving people I met on the Strip, more honest and introspective. I fostered our friendship but was careful not to encourage him too much. I didn't want to lead him on.

"Yeah, Stewart. That's the one," Shelly says, dragging me back into the present.

After she parks, we gather our backpacks and pick our way across the parking lot, gingerly stepping over broken bottles with jagged edges and half-used cigarette butts. Faint dance music emanates from the shattered windows of the hotel, but that's not our destination tonight.

"What do you know about him? Stewart, I mean," asks Shelly. There's an eager gleam in her eyes, like she can't wait to share some juicy gossip. She's always liked to know things before other people, thriving off the feeling of power it gives her.

"I know he just turned 20 and that he graduated from college early. I think he skipped some grades since he's so smart. He works for the Luxor, but I'm not sure what he does," I admit, feeling guilty. Stewart has spent hours asking me about my life, getting to know me. I'd even told him about my mom's cancer. Have I been selfish? Haven't tried as hard to learn about him?

As we wait for a blinking walk sign to turn from red to green, Shelly reveals,

"Your little buddy Stewart is the son of Johnny Stralla, the guy who owns the whole casino, the Luxor!"

"What?" I think back to my conversations with Stewart. He had told me how his mother passed away when he was a baby, an experience that made him especially sympathetic to the situation with my mom. But I can't remember him saying much about his dad.

Shelly continues, "I heard his dad is in the mob. They call him Johnny the Shark or something crazy like that. Anyway, Stewart works in the technology department. He's pretty high up there."

"What does the technology department do?" I wave to some of the other show girls on the street as we walk past. We know them all now.

"I wasn't sure either, but a guy I was talking to works security at Luxor. He told me Stewart's in charge of the computers, like the ones that do surveillance and the ones that count the money. This guy said Stewart's so smart he even invented some computer stuff, a program that can track the customers' faces or something crazy. No wonder he's such a nerd." She widens her eyes. "Did you know?"

Stunned, I answer, "I had no idea." This new information changes my perception of Stewart from a bumbling bookish man to a more calculated, tech-savvy genius. Which version of him is the real one? Also, if Stewart's dad is in the Mafia, does that mean Stewart is too? The image of shy Stewart as a gun-toting Mafioso seems ludicrous.

We reach our favorite street corner in front of New York-New York and drop our bags. Shelly puts out a hand-lettered sign we made. *Show-girl photos for $20,* it says in glitter ink surrounded by iridescent gold foil stars. The glitter had been Shelly's idea, and the stars had been mine.

She carefully balances the sign against the casino wall, angling it outward so it can be easily seen. "When he finally gets enough guts to ask you out—"

"He's not asking me out." I place a bowl for the tourists' money on the ground next to our sign. It already has a crisp $20 bill in it. We've found people are more likely to leave money if there's already some in there.

Ignoring me, Shelly continues, "When he finally asks you out, I think you should demand to go to that fancy steak place in the Luxor. He probably gets a huge employee discount there. Or…" Her eyes go wide, and she grabs my upper arm, clutching it tightly. "Maybe he even gets it for free," she whispers reverently and puts her other hand dramatically over her heart. Closing her eyes, she says, "Can you imagine it? Free steak." She licks her lips.

I laugh. "Geez. Did you skip dinner or something? Are you okay? Should I buy you a burger?"

She drops her hands back down to her side and narrows her eyes at me. "I'm serious. A girl has to eat. The guy has it bad for you, so you might as well take advantage."

I give her a doubtful look. "Stewart's nice. I wouldn't do that. Besides, you don't know if he even likes me."

Shelly doesn't bother replying. She just rolls her eyes and turns to our first customer.

41

Mom gets sicker. Her white blood cells that battle infection plummet from the chemotherapy. She gets admitted to the ICU for sepsis, sleeping for endless hours as her body struggles to fight off the bacteria in her bloodstream.

I stay by her bedside, which has a strange smell to it, roses mixed with something spicy. Almost like a man's cologne. I'm scared that if I step away for one second I might come back to find her dead. The nurses kick me out of the room, insisting that I go to the cafeteria for food or home to sleep.

Mr. Chen picks up homework from my teachers and brings it to me in the hospital. He stays with Mom when I go to school to take tests I can't delay. It's what my mom would have wanted, for me to keep up with my schoolwork as best as I can.

Mr. Chen holds me when it all becomes too much and I cry hopelessly in the hallway outside my mother's room. I don't want to cry in front of my mom, which is silly because she's unconscious. Superstitiously, I think that if I stay strong in my mother's presence it will convince her to come back to me. Like I can magically transfer my strength to her. I want to go back to the old days, twirling around the kitchen in her arms. I would do anything to keep my mother alive, even make a deal with the devil.

Miraculously, she pulls through. The antibiotics that slowly drip into her IV defeat the germs raging through her body. She opens her hazel eyes to find me sleeping in the chair beside her. My mother goes from the ICU to the regular medical floor, then to a rehabilitation hospital, and finally home.

Mr. Chen demands that Mom move into his apartment because she's too weak to climb up the stairs. He makes a bed for her in his office, with the mattress pressed up against the bent spines of his books. The musty smell of old books blends with the musty smell of sickness in the room.

Relentlessly, the medical bills keep rolling in. I sell my mom's old car. I sell our furniture and extra clothing. I let go of the apartment and move in with Mr. Chen, sleeping in the same bed as my mom and swearing I'll pay half the rent once I get more money. He refuses to accept the little bit of cash that I offer.

"Tiffany, dear, you and your mother are my family now," Mr. Chen tells me. "This is what family does. We take care of each other."

His words make me cry all over again.

42

PRESENT, ORLANDO, FLORIDA

When I see the souvenir popcorn bucket designed to look like Cinderella's carriage, I can't contain my excitement. "My favorite princess!" I exclaim, rushing over to get in line.

"I'm going to grab a pretzel. Meet you back here." Ethan walks across the street to the snack cart.

Thirty dollars poorer but happy, I munch on popcorn as I walk back to Ethan. He's bought a salted pretzel in the shape of Mickey Mouse's head, along with a cup of creamy melted cheese dip.

"That looks good." I eye his food with envy.

"Wanna trade?" He holds the salty snack out to me. "A bite of my pretzel for some of your popcorn?"

"Sure." I grasp my popcorn in one hand and take his pretzel with the other. Ethan holds the cheese dip out, so I can plunge the pretzel into it. Just before I'm going to take a bite, a rush of wind blows a piece of scarlet hair into my face. My hands full of food, I try to shake the wayward strands out of my eyes, but they remain stuck.

Ethan laughs at my predicament. "Here, let me help." He gently brushes my hair back and tucks it behind my ear.

"There you go." His smile is small and satisfied.

"Sorry." I laugh at myself. "I'm a mess."

"I don't think so." Ethan's serious now, not talking about pretzels. He leans close, his eyes never leaving mine, and says softly, "I think you're perfect. Just the way you are."

His words land like pennies tossed into a fountain. Wishes coming true.

I stare at him with my mouth hanging open, unable to form a response.

Amused by my speechlessness, Ethan grins and scoops a handful of popcorn into his mouth. "Come on, Tiffy. Let's go." He takes my hand and gently tugs me forward.

* * *

At Space Mountain I groan when I read the wait time, 90 minutes. The line snakes around the perimeter of the ride, people shifting from foot to foot.

"I heard this one's good," I tell him. "Do you mind waiting?"

He agrees, and we join the long queue. Ethan leans against the metal railing that separates us from the next portion of the line. "Cinderella is your favorite, huh?" He gestures to my bucket.

I shovel another handful of popcorn into my mouth and nod. After I swallow, I say, "I always loved the fairy godmother scene. Where Cinderella is transformed from a drab housemaid into a beautiful princess. I used to dream a fairy godmother would come and change my life like in the movie." The last sentence has a tinge of sadness.

He picks up on it. "No fairy godmother then? No one to save you?" He frowns, distressed by the idea.

"Nope." I stare at the ground, not wanting to see pity in his eyes. "Guess I learned to save myself."

The line moves forward in small increments, inch by inch. We dutifully follow the couple in front of us.

"What about happily ever after?" Ethan asks. "You read romance books. You love Disney. Surely you believe in happy endings?"

The corners of my mouth turn down. "I don't know. I've never seen happily ever after. My mom certainly didn't have it. She had me and work. She was a great mom, loved me something fierce, but I can't imagine it was the life she dreamed about when she was younger. It's hard to believe in something when you have no proof it exists."

Head tilted, I ask Ethan, "How about you? Do you believe people can have happily ever after?"

The line moves forward. He takes a deep breath. "I do, actually. My family wasn't perfect. Sometimes I didn't fit in. I was athletic, while my parents and brother were more intellectual. They had high expectations for me, and I rebelled against that. But one thing I didn't worry about was my parents' relationship. It was always solid. They have something close to happily ever after. When my brother and I were younger, we would get grossed out if my parents held hands or kissed. We'd run around screaming "eww" and pretend to gag, but inside we secretly liked it. Those gestures of affection made me feel safe. I guess that's what I mean when I say happily ever after. Having someone you can depend on. Who'll always be there for you, no matter what." Ethan blushes slightly. "I don't know. Maybe that sounds silly."

"I don't think it's silly at all. It sounds wonderful. I'd be the luckiest person to have that someday." My reassurance banishes the pink from his cheeks.

"I'm glad you had that kind of childhood," I continue, "and I'm jealous of it, if I'm being honest. I was secure knowing my mom loved me, but everything else seemed up in the air. We barely had enough money to get by. Our neighborhood was unsafe. My school wasn't the best. My mom wanted me to escape. She taught me education was the way out. So I studied hard, won scholarships, and climbed the academic ladder. I guess that's my happily ever after. To have the job I dreamed about when I was in high school. To help people when they're at their worst. I get a lot of satisfaction from work."

Ethan's eyes soften as he says gently, "That's not enough. A job is great, especially ours, but as much as you love it, a job can't love you back. It won't hold you when you get home from a hard day's work. It won't give you a pep talk when you fail. It won't wipe away your tears. You need a person for that. Someone to love you."

Quietly, I consider his words, knowing he's right. For years, decades even, I've been living half a life. Content with my job and my cat but shut off from everything and everyone else. Too scared of getting hurt, being betrayed, or, worst of all, abandoned to risk reaching out to others. Lying to myself that I don't need those kinds of personal connections. That I'm happier without them.

Spending time with Ethan in Cleveland and here at Disney World, I feel more complete than I have in a long time. I've grown accustomed to speaking out loud all the random thoughts that pop into my mind and hearing his response. It's like I'm learning to talk all over again now that he's here to listen. I don't want to go back to the silence of my old life.

As we slowly wind our way through the line, he tells me more about his family. Since I've already met Curtis, it's easy for me to picture the two of them getting into mischief. Chuckling, he tells me how his brother would pin him down like it was a WrestleMania fight, twisting his arm behind his back until he yielded. Ethan points to the scar in his left eyebrow. "Wrestling injury from my brother." Still talking, he tells me about how he would wait up late into the night, listening for the whir of the garage door to let him know his mom or dad had arrived home safely from a late shift at the hospital.

I share stories from my childhood as well. Although mine are carefully curated to leave out the bad parts, I end up telling him more than I planned. Snapshots of Mr. Chen and a young Shelly make their way into my tales. Names I haven't said in a long time. I assumed it would be sad to revisit those memories, heartbreaking to mentally dust them off, but it isn't. It's like meeting up with old friends. Things I'd forgotten suddenly come alive again—the smell of chlorine in the apartment pool, the sizzle of dumplings being pan-fried, the sensation of my mother's fingers as she ran them through my hair.

43

It's well past midnight by the time we leave the park. My eyes still have bright spots dotting my vision from where I stared too hard at the fireworks. My feet ache from walking. I'm exhausted, but it's a good kind of tired, the kind that comes from a day filled with laughter and joy.

Back at the hotel, we take the elevator up to our floor. Ethan requested his room to be close to mine, so he ended up right across the hall from me. We stop outside our hotel doors, standing apart from one another. I put one hand on the handle and stare at it, unable to look at him.

A silence falls between us. My tongue is heavy, full of things I want to say. I want to tell him how much fun I had today. How I appreciate his patience with me. How I'm hiding secrets I desperately want to reveal but can't.

That quiet stretches out until finally it breaks. Ethan steps over to me and takes my hand, not the one on the handle but the one that dangles down by my side. He tugs it, pulling me into his arms. I'm enveloped by his body, solid and warm. It's impossible not to melt into that embrace.

I tip my head up to find him peering down at me, a serious, almost painful, expression on his handsome face, like he wants to say things to me, too. Like there are a thousand words all crowding his mouth, seeking a way out.

He searches my face, and I can't hide that I'm scared, terrified of my feelings for him. Frightened that I'll disappoint him and lose him. I thought I was ready for this, but now that he's standing in front of me, my courage vanishes.

He must see my fear, because he swallows down whatever he wanted to say. Instead, he presses a soft kiss to my forehead. He bends so that his lips are right next to my ear and whispers, "Good night, Sleeping Beauty. I'll see you tomorrow." Then he lets me go, swipes his keycard, and opens his door. He stands in his doorway, looking back at me. "You go in first. I want to make sure you get in safe."

Safe.

He's always keeping me safe.

Ethan's still standing there when my door swings shut, blocking him from view. I press my hand and then my forehead against the closed door, as if I can feel him through it. I stay that way for a long time.

After I've showered and brushed my teeth, I climb into bed and pull the soft white duvet over my body. Traveling this morning and then spending the rest of the day and evening in the park has left me thoroughly depleted, but sleep evades me.

As I shift, the bedsheets tangling beneath me, I wonder, is it strength or weakness to need another person? When my mother died, and everything else happened in Las Vegas, I'd been devastated. My agony seemed like a weakness to me then. If I hadn't depended so much on Mom and others, I could have avoided all that grief. I became convinced it was better not to form attachments with other people. Better to be alone. A philosophy I've clung to for years.

Until Ethan.

Until Melanie.

Now, I'm not so sure. Which is truly the braver thing? To force people away? Or to pull them close?

Around and around, my mind goes like a hamster on a wheel. The more I think about it, the more my need for Ethan grows. It's torture, knowing he's a short hallway away from me. So close, yet a world away. I crave him, want badly to go to him, to sleep next to him like we did in Cleveland.

Trying not to overthink it, I fling off the covers, grab my hotel keycard, and cross the hallway.

I'm not running from my nightmares this time.

I'm running to him.

Ethan answers my knock immediately, like he was standing on the other side of the door.

"Can I…can I sleep with you?" I stutter, my heart fluttering as fast as a hummingbird's wings. It's frightening to be this vulnerable. To show him my glass heart, so easily shattered.

"I mean, just sleep," I clarify. "Okay? No funny business, no—what did you call it?—ravishing?"

My longing for Ethan screams at me in protest, but I tramp it down. This is all I can handle right now. I've already given up my pride by coming to his room. I'm not ready to give up anything else.

He nods, understanding, and steps aside to let me in.

I climb into his bed, noting it's still mostly made, like it hasn't been slept in. I'm guessing I wasn't the only one having a hard time going to sleep tonight. Ethan lays down next to me, and, after a brief hesitation, I slide closer and place my head on his shoulder. There's a hollow there, a dip, that fits me perfectly. As we lie together, his hand rises and he slowly runs his fingers through my hair, scalp to tip, over and over again. There's something comforting about the gesture, something familiar.

Ethan's lips are on my forehead. Not kissing, but brushing lightly across my skin. His touch sends a shiver of desire dancing down my spine. "I'm glad you knocked on my door. You belong over here."

Minutes later, I'm almost asleep, in that twilight on the threshold to oblivion, when I hear him whisper, "You belong with me."

44

PAST, LAS VEGAS, NEVADA, AGE 17

Late one night, when I'm walking back to the car with Shelly, we pass three men lounging against the wall of the Starlight. I don't pay them much attention, too distracted thinking about a trigonometry test I have the next day.

I live a double life—the dutiful daughter at home and the vixen on the Strip. Both roles are exhausting.

When I finally register the scuffing sounds of the men's footsteps behind us, a tingle of icy fear runs like cold water down my back. I shake off my distraction and focus on my surroundings. Shelly and I are on the edge of the darkened Starlight parking lot, alone with the men. The muted lights and noises from the Strip are far behind us. It's so quiet that the crunch of footsteps on the pavement and loose gravel is amplified, echoing in the night.

Shelly's hand comes out to clasp my wrist and tug me closer. She's seen the threat.

"Hey, pretty girls. Why don't you wait up?" a deep voice asks from behind.

We ignore the question, walking faster. I've been lulled into a false sense of security. Even though I work on the Strip, I've rarely been afraid. Most criminals avoid the crowded Strip because there are too many tourists as witnesses and the police are always out patrolling. Now that we're in this isolated parking lot, I see how easy it is to become prey.

Louder, with a tinge of anger, the man says, "Hey, I'm talking to you. Why don't you stop and we can have a little chat?" The rest of the men snicker as their footsteps quicken.

My heart begins to race. I refuse to look behind me, afraid that if the men see my fear they'll be like sharks scenting blood in the water. A primal voice in my mind is screaming, *danger, danger.*

Shelly's hand grips my wrist so tight it's painful, but I don't shake free. When I glance over, I see her face pulled tight. Her lips barely move when she whispers out of the corner of her mouth, "Get ready to run to the Starlight. No matter what, don't let go."

Before I can fully comprehend the instructions, Shelly cries out a sharp, "Run!" She pulls me by the wrist toward the abandoned casino side entrance where a single door sits propped open by a rock.

The first couple of steps, I stumble, thrown off by her sudden change in direction. Then I regain my footing and we are off, our legs pumping and feet pounding. We head to the doorway.

Angry exclamations from behind make me glance over my shoulder at the men pursuing us. It's a rough-looking bunch, with dirty clothing and thin limbs. Stubble covers unshaven jaws, and yellow teeth gleam as the men follow.

One man, in particular, is close behind us. In my terror, time slows down and I see with hyperintense clarity the skull and crossbones earring that dangles from his earlobe. The Skull Man pins his eyes on me with sharp focus and grins. "No point running, pretty little bird. We're going to catch you." He's not breathing hard, even though he's running.

We reach the door. For an agonizing minute, Shelly drops my wrist so we can enter single file. After we have burst into the dim hallway, we grab for each other, fumbling in the darkness until our hands find one another again. We hold on for dear life and take off.

The sound of the Skull Man slamming the door open happens seconds after Shelly drags me around a sharp corner and down a litter-strewn hallway.

"Little bird, where are you?" The man's voice echoes, bouncing off the walls. The other men's laughter follows.

Shelly leads us deeper into the first floor of the casino. We try to head up a stairwell but come to a halt because it's blocked by debris. A homeless man at the base of the stairs is passed out, not stirring as we run past.

The smell of smoke fills my nose as we rush past a room where old burn marks crawl up one wall. Another room has an empty bed frame in its center. A different room is full of chairs, stacked on one another all the way to the ceiling. We run past room after room, all dead ends.

The farther we go, the more helpless I feel. I can still hear the men behind us, getting ever closer. Skull Man calls out in a singsong mocking voice, "Come out, little bird. Come out, wherever you are."

Shelly opens a door, seemingly at random, and drags me into the room. As it closes behind us, I'm blinded, surrounded by complete darkness. I pull out my cell phone and turn on the light. We're in some sort of utility closet. Dusty boxes and old cleaning supplies are piled haphazardly along the back wall. There's no way out except for the door we just passed through.

"I'll call 911," I tell her.

"No!" she exclaims. "The police will never get here in time. Besides, how are we going to explain our clothing and the $1,000 dollars of cash in my pocket? They're going to think we're prostitutes. I don't want to get arrested." Her voice is shrill with panic.

Shelly's right. I can't go to jail. I whisper desperately, "What are we going to do, then? This door doesn't lock." I rotate the useless doorknob. The men's voices are getting closer. "They'll find us in here, eventually."

Shelly is moving boxes in the back of the room, piling them on top of each other to construct a tower. "Shut up and help me," she says curtly.

I throw my hands up in frustration. "Why? What good is that going to do?"

"We need to get up there." She points to the ceiling.

Angling my phone light up, I can just make out the shadowed edges of a rectangular depression in the ceiling. Looking closer, I realize it's a small door. The kind of hatch you use to access an attic or crawl space.

Understanding dawns on me. I quickly help Shelly place the boxes in a tall pile. We scramble up the boxes, which partially collapse under our weight, until we reach the hatch. She digs her fingers under the edge and pushes up, grunting with effort. After what seems like hours, the door pops open with a squeal. A fine rain of dust falls on our upturned faces, making us cough.

She pulls herself in, with me shoving from behind. I turn off my phone and lift my arms to be hauled up by Shelly, scraping my bare midriff as she drags me over the wooden edge. The cut burns and stings. A warm trickle runs down my belly, telling me I'm bleeding.

Silently, we let our eyes adjust to the darkness. I kick over the boxes and gently ease the door closed. The springs that control the hatch give a loud twang as it swings shut, startling me. Hopefully, those men didn't hear. We've been enclosed in a tomb, surrounded by nothing but blackness and dust. Our harsh panting fills the air. I strain to listen for clues to the men's location.

It doesn't take long before the door to the supply closet bangs open. "Oh, little bird, are you in here?" Skull Man sings into the small space.

Another man asks, "Anything?"

"Just a closet," says the Skull Man in a more normal voice.

The door closes with a rasp, and we finally release our breath.

We wait in the dark for over an hour, not wanting to use our cell phones for fear that the light might seep under the door frame and announce our location. It's pitch black. I don't know if the space we're in is large or small. I don't know what's in there with us. In the darkness, my imagination runs wild. I picture giant rats with beady red eyes. I think about all the people who have died in this hotel, of natural or unnatural causes, and how their malevolent ghosts must haunt this place. Maybe there's one next to me? Is that its clammy hand on the back of my neck or is it Shelly's breath? My fear spirals higher and higher until I might go mad.

Shelly must be feeling the same because, without warning, she leans forward and pulls the hatch door open. A rush of cool air brushes the hair away from my face. She pushes past me to topple out of our hiding spot, landing on the pile of cardboard boxes below with a stifled *hmph*. Still scared, I poke my head through the opening and whisper down to her, "Are they gone?"

"Not sure. Hang on." She cracks open the door to the hallway and peers out. "I don't see anyone."

I drop down and wince as my ankle twists underneath me. Gingerly, I rotate it to make sure I can still walk. Satisfied it's just a slight sprain, I hobble over to Shelly. "How did you know we would be safe in this room?" While we were hiding, I've been trying to figure that out.

She whispers back, "I've explored this whole place when you weren't with me. I noticed that hatch in the ceiling before, but I wasn't sure we could get it open. I didn't know where else to go."

We pause, listening at the door. I inspect myself, noting that I'm a bedraggled mess. There's a long, jagged red scrape across my belly, and dirt is embedded in my white angel outfit. Cobwebs cling to my hair.

After hearing only silence for ten long minutes, we cautiously venture into the hallway. We're paralyzed like scared rabbits, looking left and right, searching for the Skull Man and his crew. Seeing no one, we slowly make our way back to the car. At every corner and in every shadow, I'm convinced the men will jump out at us and scream, "Gotcha!" but they never do. Scrambling into our car, we hit the door lock button immediately.

We're mostly silent on the drive home. Shelly keeps checking her rearview mirror like she's scared we're being followed. Thankfully, no mysterious cars appear behind us. After dividing our money, Shelly watches from the car to make sure I safely get into Mr. Chen's apartment before she drives away.

I quickly shower and change into my pajamas in the bathroom. A smear of antibiotic ointment over my scrape makes me hiss in pain. Trying not to disturb my mom, I slide under the covers of the bed we share in Mr. Chen's old office.

Mom wakes up anyway. "Kitten? You okay?" Her voice is thick with sleep. A dry hand pats across the bed until it finds me. Feeling like a little kid, I move closer and rest my head on her bony shoulder. My mom runs long fingers through my hair, scalp to tip, over and over, like she used to do when I was young.

"I'm okay, Mama. Just glad to be home."

45

Two nights later, we're working the Strip when Rafe appears, his bulky frame vibrating with anger. I slink back, hiding partially behind Shelly, wondering what we did to make him so furious. Rafe's eyes bore into mine as he approaches. A few feet away, that murderous gaze swings to Shelly.

"Who?" he asks darkly.

Even brave Shelly blanches, but then she straightens her shoulders. "Who what?" she goads, knowing exactly what he's referring to.

I brace myself. Shelly's temper is just as bad as his.

"Who touched you?" He all but roars.

She narrows her eyes at him as she snaps, "If I'd known you'd react this way, I wouldn't have told you."

Hoping to head off an argument, I step forward. "It was some guys, three of them. No one we recognized. They didn't catch us."

"Describe them," he growls.

I do my best, limited by how dark it had been in the Starlight. The one person I can recall in frightening detail is Skull Man. His countenance is burned into my memory. The snarling curl of his lips. The sadistic gleam in his eyes. Just thinking about him makes my stomach lurch with fear.

Rafe nods once when I'm done. His voice tight like he's battling to keep control, he asks, "Are you hurt?"

"No." My hands involuntarily jump to my shirt, which covers the jagged cut spread over my entire stomach. It burns every time I move too quickly.

He tracks the movement. "Bull." He steps into my space and yanks my shirt up, exposing the wound. When he sees it, his jaw clenches so hard that I think he might crack a tooth.

He lets my shirt fall. With two short steps, he's in front of Shelly. Rafe takes her jaw in his hand, pinches her chin, and turns it side to side. "What about you? You hurt?"

"No!" Shelly jerks her head out of his reach and angrily shoves his arm away. "Stop grabbing at me."

He looks between us, pinning each of us with a hard stare, his eyes cold and merciless. "No one threatens you ever again. Neither of you. Do you hear me? Anyone who touches you is a dead man." His mouth curves into a grim smile, the edges sharp as a knife. "It won't be a quick death, either."

Rafe steps back, narrows his eyes, and jabs his finger at us one at a time. "You don't step a foot off the Strip without me. No more. I'll walk you to the car each night."

Shelly opens her mouth like she's going to argue, but he cuts her off, barking, "Not one word, Shelly. This isn't up for discussion." With that, he wheels around and stalks off, his shoulders stiff.

"Well, that was overdramatic, wasn't it?" Shelly asks, watching him leave. Her voice is steady, but the hand she raises to her forehead trembles.

* * *

A week later, Shelly passes me a crumpled newspaper article as we take our seats in history class. I smooth it with my palm and read the headline. "Three men arrested for parole violations."

A picture goes along with it. My heart bottoms out when I see the all-too-familiar faces of Skull Man and his companions. It's a mug shot, from two days ago. The men look the same with one startling difference. They've all been beaten. Skull Man has gotten the worst of it, sporting a split lip and two black eyes. He's battered, but he'll live. I can't decide how to feel about that.

Students shuffle into the room, finding their seats and chatting with each other. Another normal day for them, but not for us. I hold the article up to Shelly and whisper one word, "Rafe?"

She nods, understanding what I'm asking. The nod turns into a shrug. "Who knows for sure, though?" Class starts. I hand the article over, and Shelly buries it deep in her backpack.

46

PAST, LAS VEGAS, NEVADA, AGE 18

Rafe keeps his promise. He appears at midnight every time we leave the Strip and walks us to Shelly's car. Sometimes he strolls quietly alongside us and other times he lurks, hanging back at a distance or magically appearing a block ahead.

His presence reassures me since I doubt anyone would approach us with Rafe as our guard, but he also puts me on edge. I haven't forgotten the sensation of his rough lips on mine. Bubbles of nervous anticipation fizz through me whenever he's near. Rafe's intentions toward me remain a mystery, though. He treats me no differently than anyone else, grumpily ignoring me unless I directly address him.

When Rafe breaks his usual pattern by showing up at 10:00 p.m. instead of midnight, I know something is up. My suspicion grows even stronger when Shelly suggests the three of us get dinner at the nearby Caesars Palace food court.

Partly because it means a chance to spend more time with Rafe, I agree. Once I have my slice of greasy pizza in hand, I join Rafe and Shelly. They've selected a booth in the corner of the food court, isolated from the other diners.

Sliding onto the stiff, red pleather seat, I search their impassive faces. "What's up?"

Rafe and Shelly exchange a quick glance, and I get the impression they've carefully planned this out. The fact that they're talking behind my back sends a bitter pang of jealousy through me.

"Look," starts Shelly, "it's no secret that we all need money."

Rafe nods, remaining silent.

My eyes dart back and forth between the two of them, trying to figure out exactly where this is going. "Yeah…so?"

"So," Shelly says, with a glance at Rafe, "we found a way to get that money. Enough that all three of us won't have to worry again for a *very* long time."

"I'm not interested." I shove back, sitting deeper in the booth and crossing my arms over my chest.

"What?! We haven't even told you the plan yet." Shelly's lips purse.

I hug myself tighter and stare at the table. "You don't have to. I can already tell it involves breaking the law. I know you guys don't care about school, but I do. If I get in trouble, I can kiss my chances of getting into a good college good-bye. No one is going to accept a student with a criminal record."

Shelly reaches over to put her hand gently on my arm. She gives it a little shake. "Hey, I get it. I know what you want for your future, and I want that for you too. That's the beauty of this plan. You won't be doing anything illegal. Rafe and I will do the heavy lifting as far as that goes. We just need you to get us access. We'll take care of the rest. You won't get in trouble. Promise."

"I don't want *you* to get in trouble, either." I stare at my best friend. Most of the time, Shelly doesn't seem like she cares about her future. But I care. I picture her life five, ten years from now, and it doesn't look good.

I'm scared for her.

"We won't. This is going to be easy. Like taking candy from a baby." Now Shelly pleads, "Please, Tiffany. We really need this. I know you have all those medical bills. How're you going to pay them? How are you going to pay for college? Even if you get a scholarship, you'll need to buy other things."

I picture all the bills sitting on Mr. Chen's kitchen counter. I've organized them into three piles. A pile that needs to be paid right away, a pile that can wait for a few months, and a pile I'll never be able to afford unless I win the lottery. I think about those piles all the time, mentally shuffling them around. Trying to make them fit the amount of money in my bank account is like trying to balance a tower of Jenga blocks. If I pull out one piece, the rest of the tower will fall.

"Please," Shelly says again, with her hands clasped in front of her like she's praying. I remember this pose. It's the one she would use to get an extra popsicle for us in the summer. Thinking about our childhood brings a wave of nostalgia over me. How I long for those days, when my mom was healthy and being with Shelly had felt like home.

We used to have this locket. It said Best Friends on it and was shaped like a heart broken down the middle. I had one half of the necklace, and Shelly had the other half. We wore those necklaces until the cheap metal turned green from the chlorine in the pool and the chains broke. I still have my half. It's in the bottom of my bathroom drawer. I'll never get rid of it. I wonder if Shelly has her half, or did she throw it away once it lost its shine?

Against my better judgment, I ask, "Who's the baby you're planning to steal from?"

Another shared glance between Rafe and Shelly. "Johnny Stralla."

47

PRESENT, ORLANDO, FLORIDA

You belong with me. It echoes in my head the next day as I get ready in my room. When I'm showering. *You belong with me.* When I'm brushing my teeth. *You belong with me.* When I'm getting dressed. *You belong with me.* Did Ethan really say that last night, or had I been dreaming? What would it be like? To belong to someone? To be part of something greater than myself?

When I woke up this morning, Ethan was already gone. A note on the nightstand read:

Off to the gym.

Pick you up at 8 am for the conference.

Can't wait to go to Epcot with you today!

Ethan

The last line of the note raised a thrill through my body—excitement over Ethan or Disney or maybe both, I wasn't sure. It was hard to sort out all the strong feelings I was having this morning.

Plus, how cute is it that Ethan had signed his name? Like, who else would leave notes next to my sleeping head? A silly smitten smile broke out whenever I thought of that signature. He is adorable *and* hot. Like catnip for women.

A knock on my hotel door is followed by Ethan calling through it, "Tiffy? You alive in there? We gotta get going before registration closes."

"Coming," I yell back.

When I step out of the bathroom, a cloud of steam and perfume follows. I've made sure to look extra nice today, curling my hair until it falls into smooth shiny waves away from my face and taking time to get my makeup just right. I'm wearing a form-fitting gray pencil skirt and an ivory blouse with low black heels to complete my ensemble. It's professional with a feminine kick. A sexy librarian look was my goal.

"Ready," I sing out and open the door to let him in. I sashay across the room to get my purse, feeling kind of proud of myself. I'm not normally a sashaying kind of woman.

It's satisfying to see Ethan's eyes widen and to hear him say, "You look nice. All those khaki-wearing radiologists downstairs won't be able to concentrate on the many causes of cardiomegaly with you around."

Suddenly self-conscious, I clutch my chest. "Is it too much? I can change." I'm about to wheel around and sprint back into the bathroom when Ethan hastily says, "No. No. You're perfect. This conference just got a whole lot more interesting, is all."

His appreciative gaze rakes over my body, so heavy it's as if he's just reached out and caressed me. The slow, sexy smile he gives me lets me know he likes what he sees.

"Come on, then. Let's go. We wouldn't want to keep them waiting." I bat my eyelashes and deliberately brush my arm against his as I walk by, enjoying the way it makes Ethan suck in his breath. It's been a long time since I flirted. Those skills are so rusty they're almost nonexistent, but today I might refresh them.

48

Ethan and I join the long line that leads to the registration table. After I'm signed in, the registration woman hands me an ID badge. It hangs on a long red lanyard. I turn it over in my hands, inspecting it.

American College of Advanced Radiology (ACAR)
22nd Annual Conference

Dr. Tiffany Hart

Columbus, OH

An extra green ribbon along the bottom says, *Guest Speaker*. It's only given to doctors who are giving lectures. I slip the lanyard over my head and take in my surroundings. We're in the conference area of the hotel. A wide lobby has beige carpet and paneled walls. Plump leather club chairs with small end tables line the room.

Other doctors, mostly dressed in khaki just as Ethan predicted, mill around chatting with each other or cluster around the breakfast buffet. This is one of the largest annual radiology conferences, so the lectures will be held in the hotel's main ballroom. Large wooden double doors stand open, offering a view of the room filled with rows of uncomfortable-looking chairs.

Before we go in, I want breakfast and coffee. Ethan places his matching red lanyard over his head, messing up his hair. I almost reach up to smooth down the unruly spikes but catch myself at the last minute. "Want to see what they have to eat?"

"Yes, please. I'm starving." Ethan heads to the buffet, his long legs eating up the distance between him and the food.

"You're *always* hungry," I say with an affectionate eye roll as I follow him.

The breakfast is spread over a long table covered with a white tablecloth. Baskets of appetizing pastries, toast, and bagels are interspersed with bowls of fresh fruit and yogurt. At the end of the table is a self-service coffee bar.

I choose a chocolate croissant and make a cup of coffee. I'm adding in three packets of sugar when Ethan catches up to me.

"Are you going to survive without your favorite coffee this morning?" Ethan teases as he hands me an extra packet of sugar, which I gladly accept.

"Don't kid yourself. We're totally going to a real coffee shop later." I swirl the coffee and sugar together with a small wooden stir stick, thinking about how nice it is to be with someone who knows you, who remembers all your little quirks and preferences.

"Of course we are," Ethan agrees affably, balancing his overloaded plate in his hand. He has so much food piled up that it looks like he took one of each item.

Gingerly biting into my chocolate croissant, I ask, "Did you do your Karate Kid routine at the gym this morning?" I wipe a spot of chocolate filling off the corner of my mouth with my napkin. Ethan's eyes follow the movement and linger on my lips. I notice where he's looking and remind myself that I want to work on my flirting skills today. To test my power, I use the tip of my tongue to lick the rest of the chocolate off. His eyes darken at the sight.

Ethan drags his gaze away from my mouth. "Yeah, I did my usual morning warmup."

"Must have been quite the show. I'm sure everyone at the gym enjoyed seeing that." I'm trying to tease him, but picturing Ethan so tall, and handsome as hell, stretching out his long, lean body in the gym makes my voice come out low and raspy. My breathing has sped up. I'm not thinking about the over 100 other radiologists at the conference.

All I can think of is him.

"I don't remember you complaining about it," Ethan says with a smoldering look. He steps closer to me. So close that I can see the rise and fall of his chest as his breath quickens. The way his full lips part with a soft exhale and his eyes grow heavy-lidded as they stare down at me.

We're standing in the middle of the lobby, staring hungrily at each other. *Geez.*

I pull at the neckline of my blouse, suddenly overheated. I'm trying to seduce Ethan, but now *I'm* the one hot and bothered. A chiming bell sound rings out, signaling the beginning of the conference. People start moving into the ballroom.

Hoping that the burning flush on my cheeks isn't too noticeable, I take Ethan's hand and pull him toward the room. "Come on. Let's go find a seat."

He intertwines his fingers into mine, startling me, but I don't pull away.

That's how we walk into the conference together.

Holding hands.

49

PAST, LAS VEGAS, NEVADA, AGE 18

"Johnny Stralla?! That's who you want to steal from? Are you crazy? The owner of the Luxor? No way." I look from Shelly to Rafe with my mouth hanging open in shock. "We can't do that. We're just a couple of kids. You think we can outsmart a man who is reportedly a mob boss? That's sheer lunacy."

"Not all of us have a mom like yours, Tiffany." Shelly can't hide the bitterness in her voice. "We've been taking care of ourselves for as long as we can remember. We aren't kids. I don't think we've *ever* been kids. We haven't had that luxury."

"Well, it doesn't matter. There's still no way we can get past Johnny Stralla. I can't believe I'm sitting here listening to this." I put my fingertips to my temples, rubbing where a stress headache is growing.

Rafe breaks his silence. He holds up his hand as if to quiet me. In a low voice, he says, "Calm down. Stralla will never know it was us."

Incredulous, I ask, "Oh yeah? How exactly will that work?"

He leans back casually, unruffled by my agitation. "Because we'll be wearing masks."

"Well, I'm pretty sure that once he sees you wearing a mask, he's going to know that you're there to rob him," I say sarcastically.

A satisfied smirk lifts Rafe's mouth. "Not if *he* asks us to wear the masks."

"And why would he do that?" I demand, outraged that we're having this conversation.

Rafe pulls a yellow piece of paper that, judging by its dingy creases, has been folded and refolded many times, out of his back pocket. He wordlessly slides it across the table to me.

I carefully unfold and examine the paper. It's a photocopy of a smaller invitation that reads:

You are cordially invited to the 13th annual
black and white masquerade ball

Hosted by John Stralla at his home

3900 Las Vegas Blvd., Tower One

The Penthouse

I drop the paper back onto the crumb-dusted tabletop. "How are you planning on getting into this party? I'm guessing you weren't invited."

Eyes gleaming, Shelly excitedly leans toward me. "That's where you come in."

"Me?" I question, pointing a finger at myself.

"You're our ticket to get through that door." Shelly's hand has returned to my arm like she wants to hold me in place.

A disbelieving laugh escapes me. "How? I wasn't invited either."

"I know, but Stewart was. He goes every year." Shelly pins me with a pleading stare.

I have a powerful urge to walk away. To stand up and march right out of there, never talking to these people again. But the thought of my mother's medical bills and the lack of money to pay them keeps me seated.

"Let me guess—you want me to get Stewart to take me to that ball?"

Rafe gives me an approving look. "Smart girl. There's a reason you're going to be valedictorian."

"Then what? Say I get Stewart to take me. What happens then?" I feel like I'm on a roller coaster, a big and scary one. I want to get off, but I'm already strapped in and at the top, waiting for the stomach-jolting drop back down to the ground.

Rafe takes over, eager to share his strategy. "Johnny Stralla has a safe in his home office. It's full of everything we need: cash, diamonds, casino chips, you name it. The best part is that it's his personal stash, so he's made sure it's all stuff that can't be traced."

He grins, a reckless shine in his eyes. "The room is protected by a lock on the wall. It's the kind that's activated by a specially coded badge, you know, one of those plastic keycards you see all the employees wearing. Once you get to the party with Stewart, we need you to lift that keycard off him. It'll have access to the highest security locations, including the office door. Just give the card to us. I know the code for the safe. We'll take care of the rest."

Shelly joins in, eager to convince me. "See, Tiffany? You won't be at risk. At the very worst, you get caught trying to steal the keycard. You can easily pretend it was a mistake and play it off. Stewart has a big-time crush on you. He'll believe anything you say. If you can't get the keycard, the whole deal is a bust, which will suck, but we won't be any worse off than we are now. If you do get it, everything changes for us. You can pay off those bills, and I can move out of my mom's house."

I turn to Rafe and ask, "What about you? What would you do with the money?"

There's a haunted expression on his face. "Me? I'd get as far away from here as I can."

"Really?" I frown, unhappy with his response. I don't want Rafe to leave. The thought of never seeing him again settles heavily in my heart, a boulder sinking to the ocean floor.

Hollow-eyed, he nods.

"How do you know all of this? About the ball, the office, the safe?" My brows rise, questioning.

Shelly dismissively waves her hand. "Rafe knows people. He hears things."

I'm unconvinced. "What people?" I ask him. "How do we know if they're telling the truth?"

"It's the truth," he answers without hesitation. "The code to the safe is legit. I've triple-checked it myself. I can get Shelly and me into the party, and I can open the safe. The only thing I don't have access to is that office. The keycard is too heavily encrypted. We need Stewart's badge. It's the only way."

I shake my head, my hands tightening into fists. "I don't believe you. Who would have that kind of knowledge? It's too far-fetched."

Rafe scrubs a hand over his face and sighs heavily. "We have people all over this city. You wouldn't believe the kind of information we have access to."

"We?" I raise my hands palms up, frustrated by his vague response. If they want me to help, I'm going to need better answers than this.

"My family." His eyes shift to the left, and there's something odd in his expression. Is that guilt? Shame? I've never seen Rafe unable to stare someone down.

"What about cameras? Security?" I swallow the last bite of my pizza, not even tasting it.

"All controlled from that office with Stewart's keycard." Before I can ask another question, Rafe looks at me, *really* looks at me. The full force of his laser-eyed focus makes me catch my breath. *This* is what I've been wanting. His attention.

"Tiffany, I *promise* you. I can do this. I can pull it off, but not alone. Not without your help."

It's hard to deny him when he's staring at me like that, like he's on a sinking ship and I'm the only one holding a life preserver. My resolve wavers. "Who knows if I can even get Stewart to take me? He's never mentioned this party." I stand and gather my trash. The pizza I ate has turned into a lead ball in my stomach.

Shelly piles her dirty plate and napkin on her plastic tray. "That's step one. Let's see if you can get him to take you. You can decide what you're comfortable with after that. Okay?"

I'm aware that she's luring me deeper into their plan by giving me the illusion of choice. It's too late for that. The roller coaster has already started down the hill, and the pit of dread in my belly tells me that I'm on it for the entire ride.

50

Getting Stewart to invite me to the ball turns out to be incredibly easy. Just a couple of well-placed hints and he brings it up like it's his own idea. He tells me that he hates these parties because he feels awkward and he usually hides in the bathroom, waiting for the event to be over. He's relieved when I agree to go with him, acting like *I'm* the one doing him a favor.

The subterfuge makes me feel terrible. I picture myself as Pennywise the Clown about to drag Stewart down into the sewers and devour him. *This is for Mom,* I remind myself daily. If I can't keep paying the medical bills, then she won't get the treatment she needs.

The day before the party, we head to the Strip in our show-girl costumes. Today, Shelly drives a red SUV with a dented bumper. Her hair is a rich brunette, all her usual bright colors gone. The new hair color is for the heist. She doesn't want to stand out in the crowd in case we're pursued, a thought that terrifies me.

"You think we can really pull this off?" I ask. The car window is open, and the warm desert wind whips my hair, sending strands into my eyes. I comb them aside with my fingers, holding my hair to the side in a loose ponytail.

"Oh, yeah. With the information Rafe has, we'll get that money," Shelly answers without hesitation.

"How can you be so sure? How does Rafe know so much about Johnny?" My mind swirls with unanswered questions.

She shoots me an incredulous look. "Even after everything that happened with those guys who chased us, you still don't know?"

"Know what?" I lift my hands, palms up.

Shelly shakes her head. "Who Rafe is."

For a minute, I almost don't want to know. I want to hold onto my dream version of Rafe, the one with the secret heart of gold. But now that we're planning this robbery, it's time to let that illusion go. I need to understand what I'm getting into. "What do you mean?"

Shelly gives me a look of affectionate disgust. "This is what you get for always having your head stuck in a book, Tiffany. I swear an alien spaceship could land in the middle of school and you wouldn't even notice." Her smile softens her words.

"Rafe is part of the Kingsman Gang, their Latin branch. His whole family is involved, with his dad as the head. I don't know all the details, just that he's high up and not only because he's related. You should hear what people say about him, that they've never seen someone that young shoot up the ranks so fast. They talk about how he's so smart. So ruthless. I think his dad is grooming him to take over." She's somber, almost sad, as her eyes meet mine. "He's their future."

"Oh." It's what I expected, but the thought of organized crime makes me cringe. I can't believe that I'm consorting with an actual gang.

God help me.

"That's why Rafe used to have bruises on his arms? From gang stuff?" I ask.

Shelly shifts uncomfortably in her seat. "That or else from his dad. I hear he's a real asshole."

"What about Rafe's mom?" There's a lump in my throat from the thought that Rafe was abused. My fantasy reoccurs, the one where I rescue him.

Shelly sighs and rubs the bridge of her nose. "What mom? He's never had one. I don't know what happened to her, though. No one talks about it."

"I don't get it." I frown, working through this new information. "You said Rafe's their future, but he said he wants to leave. Won't his family be mad?"

"They'll be furious." Her fear is palpable, which in turn scares me. I've seen Shelly mad plenty of times but hardly ever frightened. "If Rafe stays," she says and swallows, "he'll end up dead or in jail. He might be their future, but that's the only future left to him."

We're silent then, each of us lost in our thoughts. Palm trees sway outside the car window. Wind blows dust across an empty lot. A mangy dog prowls down an alleyway.

"What're you going to wear to the party, Tiffany?" Shelly interrupts the quiet, and I swing my head back to her.

I perk up, excited to share my idea. "My mom has this old dress. She keeps it in the very back of her closet. It's beautiful, pure white with a long full skirt. Super fancy. It even has these deep pockets that'll be perfect for hiding the keycard." I've wanted to try that dress on since I was a child, but Mom never let me. Plus, it was always too big. I've grown as tall as my mother, so it should fit.

"What? Like a wedding dress?" Shelly asks, with a side glance my way.

"No, more like a ball gown." That fabric had felt so smooth in my hands when I touched it as a small child. I've never forgotten the sensation.

She tilts her head. "Why would your mom have a dress like that?" The blinker makes a clicking noise as we take a right at the next intersection.

"Not sure. I've never seen her wear it. When I asked about it, she changed the subject." I adjust the straps of my bikini top. They're digging into my shoulders again. I'll have red grooves in my skin by the end of the night.

"If she doesn't talk about the dress, why didn't she throw it away?" Shelly pulls into the Starlight parking lot.

After she parks, we look around carefully before unlocking our doors and stepping out of the SUV. We're both still gun-shy after our run-in with Skull Man. This parking lot stirs those dark memories.

"I have no idea where that dress comes from. My mom has secrets, a whole life before we moved here that she won't talk about. It's frustrating because it's my history too. I should have some right to it. I don't know where or who I come from." Tears prick at the back of my throat. The stress of the upcoming ball, not to mention school and my mom's illness, is making me overly emotional. I've been on the verge of a meltdown several times this past week.

Shelly sees my distress. "Hey," she says gently, "don't feel too bad about it.

I know exactly who and where I come from. Let me tell you, it's no comfort. More like a self-fulfilling prophecy. You're lucky not to have all that baggage weighing you down."

I blink back my tears before they fall. "It's just hard sometimes, like I can't really know who I am since I don't know where I come from."

Shelly reaches an arm around my shoulder and gives me a soft squeeze. "I know who you are. You're Tiffany, the best friend and daughter anyone could ever ask for. You're smart and brave and hot as hell." She lightly pinches my arm and grins mischievously at the last part.

"Don't you ever forget those things." Shelly's demeanor changes. Her eyes glisten, and she chokes out fiercely, "No matter what happens after tomorrow, don't forget who you are and that I love you." She's not usually big on public displays of affection, so I'm shocked when she pulls me into a long, hard hug.

Looks like I'm not the only one worried about the robbery.

"I love you too, Shelly." I hold my best friend tight, my tears forgotten.

51

After the taxi drops me off at the entrance to the Luxor, I pause to look up at the pyramid-shaped structure. The smoky glass walls of the hotel angle steeply upward until they meet at a sharp peak at the very top of the building, where a blinding column of light shoots straight up, illuminating the night sky.

Dark creatures flap in and out of this beam of light, like ancient fire-breathing dragons. *Bats,* I realize with a start. The moon is a tiny fingernail of silver in the distance.

I feel eyes on me, but when I turn no one's looking my way. *Weird.* Probably just overthinking things since I'm stressed. I run shaky hands over the shimmering white satin of my dress, taking comfort from its cool silkiness. The sleeveless bodice shows off my long creamy neckline and the soft hollow between my breasts. The dress fits like a glove. There's no way it could fit so well if it hadn't been made for my mother.

Earlier, when I was getting dressed, I had unzipped the garment bag that held the dress, and a faint scent of flowers and perfume, decades-old like a distant memory, wafted out. Again, I wonder when my mother wore it last.

Right before I left my room, I had glanced at my smudged full-length mirror and had frozen, staring at my reflection. I look good in this white dress. I won't use the word beautiful. My mother is beautiful. I'm a poor imitation of that, like a faded print when the copy machine runs out of ink. But in this dress, with my hair and makeup done, I can admit that I'm pretty.

I suck in one last breath of the crisp night air and head inside to find Stewart in the hotel lobby. We've arranged to meet there so he can escort me up to the party. "I'll have to get you past all the security," he had told me earlier, which made my heart constrict with fear.

When Stewart sees me for the first time across the crowded lobby, his mouth drops open. His obvious admiration fuels my confidence. I walk slowly to him with my head held high.

Cheeks turning red, he stutters, "Wow, Tiffany, you look…gorgeous. I'm going to be the…the envy of every other man in the room tonight. I can't wait to show you off."

Now it's my turn to blush. "Thanks, Stewart, that's nice of you to say."

Traitor, my mind screams, *you're going to break his heart*. I shove the intrusive thoughts away. If I'm going to play my role this evening, I can't afford to be distracted by my conscience.

Stewart sticks out his elbow and says, "Shall we?"

Like a scene in a glamorous Hollywood movie, I loop my arm through his and say, "We shall."

He leads me to a single elevator in the back corner of the lobby, partially hidden by large potted palm trees. It has golden doors with an ornate scrolling pattern. There's no button to push, just a small square metal plate with a sign above it that reads Private.

Using his free hand, Stewart digs in his front pants pocket. He produces a rectangular plastic badge that has his picture and name on it. I go rigid when I see the keycard in his hand.

That's it. That's what I need to steal from him tonight.

Seeing it makes everything real. If I take it from him, there will be no going back to who I was before. That person will be gone, dead to me. I'll cross a threshold and become a criminal. Someone willing to sacrifice innocents like Stewart for my own needs.

Do I want to be that person? Do I have any choice?

When he places the keycard over the metal plate next to the door, a chime sounds and the elevator whirs to life. Soon it arrives, and we step inside. A subtle jolt of the floor tells me we're in motion, although the ride is incredibly smooth.

"Is it true this elevator is actually going sideways because of the building's pyramid shape?" I ask, trying to distract Stewart with small talk as I carefully watch him return the keycard into the same front pocket.

With a restrained laugh, Stewart says, "Not sideways. It's on an incline… a 39-degree angle, but so subtle you can't really feel it. If you're being technical, they aren't actually elevators. They're called…called inclinators."

The inclinator doors ding open, and a long hallway with polished marble floors stretches in front of us. The walls are papered with shiny gold wallpaper. Large mirrors are set into the ceiling. It's disorienting to see an upside-down version of myself when I look up.

A door labeled "stairs" is located to the right of the elevator, a green exit sign glowing above it. I mark it in my mind.

We step into the hallway, and Stewart says, "Oh, almost forgot." He drops my arm to reach into his opposite pants pocket and pull out a black fabric mask. He puts it on, covering the skin around his eyes, but leaving his nose and mouth exposed.

I retrieve a similar mask from my purse. My mask is made of white lace that I hand-sewed with Shelly's help. A thin band of elastic holds it tight over my eyes.

It's funny how a small scrap of fabric can make such a big difference in a person's appearance. Stewart looks almost like a dashing pirate with his mask and tailored three-piece suit. He watches me adjust my mask until it fits comfortably. His bashful gaze hangs on me a little too long. Guilt twists my insides, sharp and painful.

A short line of people are waiting to walk through a metal detector manned by a burly man wearing a dark suit. When it's our turn, I notice a bulge under the man's jacket that looks suspiciously gun-shaped. I gulp down my fear.

A stunning black woman stands just past the guard, checking sheets of paper clutched in her hands. A thin wire extends up her neck to an earpiece, which she occasionally touches, pushing it closer and frowning as she listens. When we approach, she drops her hand from her ear.

"Stewart," the woman says warmly. "How lovely to see you, and you've brought a date." The way her honey-colored eyes light up confirms what I already know, that Stewart doesn't usually attend these events with a woman.

She looks me over approvingly and says, "My, aren't you lovely?" I flush at the compliment. I'm about to respond, but Stewart jumps in and answers, "Thanks, Irene." He says it like he's personally responsible for my beauty. He preens at my side, standing straighter and more confident than I've ever seen before.

Irene nods regally. "Your father is already inside." She gestures to a set of double doors with the same metal plate on the wall beside them.

Stewart scans his keycard once more, and the doors swing open. I walk into the most gorgeous room. It has a massive sunken living room, grounded by the same marble floor as in the hallway outside and surrounded by soaring floor-to-ceiling windows. There are no curtains to impede the view. The twinkling lights of the world-famous Las Vegas Strip spread out before us in breathtaking glory. We're so high up that I can see the rooftop pools and bars of the smaller hotels.

A string quartet plays quietly in the corner of the room. The buzz of lively conversation fills gaps in the music. Model-perfect waitresses circulate, holding silver platters of champagne and appetizers. When a masked waitress stops before us, Stewart takes two bubbling flutes from her tray and hands one to me. "Cheers," he says, gently clinking his glass against mine.

"Cheers," I echo halfheartedly. I hesitate before I bring the drink to my lips. When I drank alcohol before, at the Starlight party, it had been in the dark with a bunch of kids my age. Now, out in the open and surrounded by adults, it feels wrong. I worry I'll get in trouble, which is ridiculous because of all the laws I'm here to break tonight, underage drinking is the least of them. I tell myself to stop being silly and take a small sip, letting the bubbles fizz in my mouth before swallowing it down.

My gaze wanders, and I'm immediately overwhelmed by the elegance in this room. I had thought my mom's dress is beautiful, but it pales next to the beaded gowns glittering before me. Fancy gold watches and diamond-studded cufflinks on the men's wrists reflect light back into my eyes.

The scene is even more surreal because everyone is wearing a mask. Some only cover the wearer's eyes while others cover half of or the entire face. Elaborate feathered and sequined masks make my homemade one look cheap by comparison. The sheer opulence of the setting leaves me feeling small and unworthy.

Sensing my hesitation, Stewart leans toward me and whispers, "You look beautiful."

I shoot him a grateful smile, paired with another stab of guilt.

"Come on. I want you to meet someone." Stewart takes my hand and leads me through the crowd. We make our way past clusters of people talking and drinking. I stare at the floor, scared to step on any of the exquisite dresses with skirts so long they puddle on the marble.

I almost bump into Stewart when he stops before a small group of partygoers clustered around a thin man with dark hair and sharp brown eyes. The man is about my mom's age. He's impeccably dressed in an expensive-looking black tuxedo.

Once the crowd clears, Stewart steps forward, still holding my hand. "Dad, this is Tiffany." Stewart beams proudly at me.

The man reaches out to shake my hand. His grasp is almost painfully firm. "Tiffany, nice to meet you. I'm John Stralla. Glad you could make it to the party."

Johnny Stralla, the owner of this penthouse, of this whole hotel and casino. Johnny Stralla, who, if rumors are to be believed, is also called Johnny the Shark with ties to the Mafia in New York and Chicago. A man who owns numerous businesses throughout the city, some legal and some not. Drugs, guns, and who knows what else supposedly filter through his shadier establishments. I shift uncomfortably, thinking about how this is the man that Shelly and Rafe plan to rob. He doesn't seem like the kind of guy anyone should mess with.

We're in over our heads.

"Um, hello. Thank you for having me. Your home is gorgeous." I keep my grip firm as I return his handshake.

His easy smile doesn't match the coldness in his eyes. "Of course. Please make yourself at home—" Johnny freezes, his gaze on my dress. It lingers there for seconds that stretch into minutes. His eyes snap up and search my face, looking puzzled. "Beautiful gown," he says slowly, then trails off. He gives his head a shake, like he's waking up. Before I can give his odd behavior much thought, he abruptly changes the topic, his expression warming as he looks at Stewart. "My son has told me what a brilliant student you are, Tiffany. Have you given any thought to where you'd like to attend college?"

The fact that Stewart has been talking about me to his dad is a shock. I don't think of myself as important enough to warrant their attention. "Honestly, I'll go wherever I get the best scholarship." I glance away, embarrassed to discuss my poverty with someone so rich and powerful.

Just then, a large man with an earpiece approaches Stewart and whispers in his ear. Stewart frowns. "Tiffany, can you excuse me for a minute? They're having problems with one of the gaming computer systems downstairs. It's frozen, and they need me to access the administration software to fix it. I'll just be gone a minute."

Not understanding half of the computer jargon Stewart used, I nod. He quickly squeezes my elbow and then he's gone, leaving me alone with his dad.

Feeling his eyes on me, I meet Johnny's narrowed gaze. "If you are planning to stay in Nevada, I have some connections at the university. I could make a few phone calls—if you want, that is." His eyes slide over to the empty spot that Stewart just occupied. Shocked, I realize that he's trying to bribe me to date Stewart by dangling admission to college.

He continues coldly, "Or I could make the same phone calls and guarantee that you don't get into any college." I can see why he's called the shark now. His eyes are black and bottomless. There is no emotion in them, only cunning.

His threat infuriates me. I'm already stretched tight with tension this evening. Johnny's words provoke me, bringing on a quiet, fiery rage. My hands clench into fists by my side. "You would do that? Take away my only real chance for a future?" My eyes shoot daggers at him. I'm walking a thin line between my anger and the need to control it for Rafe's and Shelly's sake. "You must really care about Stewart to say that."

There's a flicker of surprise, maybe even admiration, at my reaction. Clearly, Johnny's not used to people talking back to him.

His expression neutral, he says, "It's true. I do care about Stewart. I also care about my business. My son is integral to running my casino successfully.

I won't have him distracted like a heartsick puppy." Johnny's look grows distant. "I'm going to need Stewart's full focus over these next couple of years."

I'm about to respond when our conversation is interrupted by Stewart's return.

Sensing the tension in the air, Stewart asks, "You okay, Tiffany?" His face puckers with concern, his brown eyes bouncing back and forth between his dad and me.

My smile is bright, but false. "I'm fine." Deliberately, I angle my body away from Johnny. I don't want to talk to him anymore. Maybe he deserves to have his money stolen.

Without a clear thought in my head, I wrap my arms around Stewart and hug him, putting my back to Johnny. As I draw Stewart close, my hand slips into his front pocket and retrieves the slick plastic keycard. "Did you get everything fixed?" I ask as I pull out of the embrace.

A happy smile crosses Stewart's face. "All good now."

Johnny stares at me suspiciously before he excuses himself with a nod of his head and a "Nice to meet you."

I don't respond to him, still silently fuming as I slide the keycard deep into my pocket. I'll fight for my mom and my future, even if that means taking on Johnny the Shark.

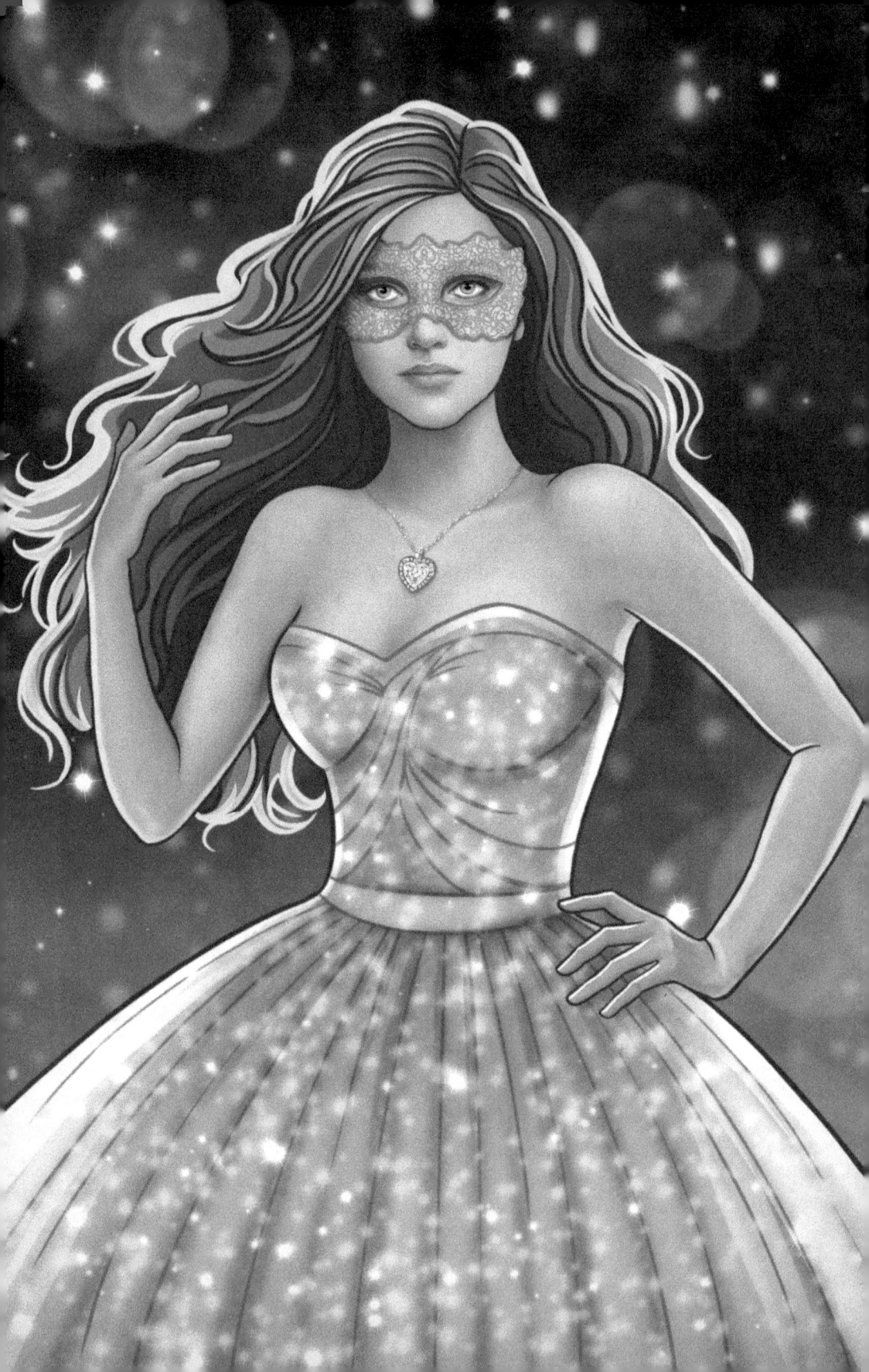

52

I savor the bubbles that tickle across my tongue from the champagne. It makes me recall that night at the Starlight, the sour taste of the strawberry wine. The sweet taste of Rafe's mouth rough against mine. Thinking about Rafe must magically conjure him because I look up to see his masked emerald eyes staring at me from across the room. I do a double take, doubting for a moment that he's real.

Rafe is transformed, wearing a black tuxedo with his normally unruly hair slicked away from his face. He is clean-shaven, his usual stubble removed to reveal a sharp, angled jaw. He's breathtaking…and he shouldn't be here. Not yet anyway. With a false smile for Stewart, I ask him to hold my glass while I use the restroom. I snake my way through the crowd, searching the sea of unfamiliar faces.

Nothing.

Rafe has disappeared.

In the hallway that leads to the bathroom, I almost shriek when a cold-fingered hand grabs my arm and pulls me into an open bedroom. Rafe kicks the door closed. We're locked away, alone together. His presence fills the room, menacing and sexy all rolled into one.

"What are you doing here?" I ask breathlessly, followed immediately by, "Is Shelly okay?" I look behind him at the empty room, almost expecting to see her there. "You aren't supposed to get here until midnight."

Rafe sits down on the edge of the bed, leaving me awkwardly standing above him. He leans back on his elbows, eyes lazily roving over me. "You look pretty tonight."

"Rafe," I warn, wanting answers.

A devilish smile curls one corner of his mouth. "Shelly's still coming at midnight."

"But what are *you* doing here?" I sit down on the bed next to him, keeping a distance. I don't want to be distracted right now. Not with so much at stake.

Rafe sits up straight, matching my posture. "I was invited at the last minute." Seeing my glare of annoyance, he explains. "Just got here. Didn't have time to tell you in advance." He stares at me, carefully considering his next words. "You know my work?"

I nod silently.

"The main dealer Johnny the Shark uses had an unexpected…complication and couldn't make it to the party. They brought me here instead. I'll supply the partygoers with everything they need. Don't be fooled. There's a lot more than just alcohol flowing tonight." Rafe clasps his hands loosely in his lap, completely relaxed.

I regard him suspiciously. "What complication?"

Shrugging nonchalantly, he says, "An anonymous tip made the police take him into custody. He should get out in, oh…three to five years." Again, the devil's grin.

Johnny isn't the only shark at this party tonight. Apparently, I'm a minnow swimming in a sea of them.

"I was going to be here later, anyway. Better to come early so I can keep an eye on you." His voice is low and husky, sending a thrill through me. Rafe slides closer to me on the bed. His proximity sparks a fire that burns quickly through my body. He runs a finger lightly down my bare arm. Goosebumps rise, marking the trail of his touch. His eyes glitter like diamonds in the moonlight that shines through the window. I shiver, hot and cold all at once.

"How do I look? Like I fit in? Like I belong?" he asks like it's a game of truth or dare and I picked truth.

I take in his black tuxedo jacket and note the way it hugs the muscles of his shoulders and upper arms. Shelly was right. He must be working out more, or maybe he's growing. I forget we're still young sometimes. He graduated last year, so he must be what? Nineteen now? I recently turned 18. Both of us are old enough to be tried as adults if we get caught, a most terrifying thought.

"You look so…different," I answer honestly. "I've never seen you like this before."

Rafe's finger stops its caress, its owner displeased by my response. "Yeah, well, gotta fit in. You know, a wolf in sheep's clothing, isn't that what they say?" He stands up from the bed and moves to gaze out the window, his stiff back to me.

I've hurt his feelings somehow, but I'm not sure what he wanted to hear. Struggling to regain his attention, I say, "You look nice, very handsome." It doesn't matter now. The moment is gone. His eyes are shuttered when he walks back from the window. Whatever light had glowed in them a moment ago has been snuffed out.

"Do you have it?" Rafe asks flatly.

Flushed, feeling rejected, I dig Stewart's keycard out of my pocket and hand it over. Faster than my eyes can follow, he makes it disappear.

"Better get back out there before he misses you." Rafe doesn't bother to say who "he" is. We both know. I go to the door and twist the knob. As I peer out to make sure the coast is clear, he whispers in my ear, "Stick to the plan." My body involuntarily shudders at the feeling of his warm breath on the back of my neck. He moves quietly, a cat on soft fur paws. I hadn't realized he was so close. Rafe's burning hand is on the small of my back as he gently pushes me out into the hallway. The soft click of the door tells me that he's closed it, locking himself in the room, away from me.

53

I return to the party. The crowd's mood has shifted while I was gone. The music is louder now. The string instruments have been replaced by a headphone-wearing DJ who bops to the beat as he works the turntables. Guests surge and vibrate on a dance floor, pressed up against the wall of windows.

With Rafe's words echoing in my mind, I notice details that had previously escaped me. Partygoers are sprawled across plush couches, their limbs akimbo and eyes dilated. There is a layer of debauchery here, buried beneath the elegant surface.

Stewart's waiting where I left him. "I thought you'd gotten lost," he jokes and hands me back my half-drunk glass of champagne.

"Just fixing my makeup." I take a sip of my bubbly drink, letting the alcohol warm me. It's scary how easily the lies come, but then again, I've had lots of practice over the last few months lying to my mom and Mr. Chen. Telling them I'm out studying when I'm actually taking photos on the Strip. Hiding wads of cash in my school backpack until I can deposit it in the bank.

Pointing toward the dance floor, Stewart asks, "Do you want to dance?"

Dancing is one of my least favorite activities. I'm all awkward elbows and knees, never quite sure what to do with my hands. The only dancing I've ever enjoyed was in the isolation of Shelly's room when we were young and would dance wildly to the latest boy-band hit.

"No, thanks. I'm a terrible dancer."

Stewart lets out a puff of air. "Thank goodness. I loathe dancing. I'm not sure why I asked. I didn't want you to feel like you're missing out on anything tonight because of me."

He's kind, this man. I wish for a moment that he wasn't. It makes me more of a monster.

"I don't think that," I reassure him.

As I gaze around the room, I notice expensive-looking paintings and statues placed in alcoves along the walls. Artfully placed lighting highlights each one. "Those are gorgeous pieces of art. Does your dad collect them?" I move closer to examine a painting of yellow and orange poppy flowers in a brown vase. It almost looks like a Van Gogh.

"He does but not because he appreciates their beauty. He sees them as another way to diversify his portfolio."

I sense this is a point of contention between Stewart and his father. "How do *you* see them?"

After a moment of thought, he says, "When I look at my father's artwork, I think of the men and women who made it. How talented they must have been. I always wonder if it was hard for them. To make something so beautiful, to pour their heart and soul into it, only to have to sell it away. Hand it off to someone who might not value it the same way they did." A side glance at me, as he adds, "It must be hard to lose something you love."

How he says love makes me uncomfortable. There's too much weight on that word. My eyes scan the room, on the lookout for Rafe or Shelly. I see neither one.

"You didn't mention that you're Johnny Stralla's son when we first met," I blurt, trying not to sound accusatory, but I've been wondering why he never brought it up.

"It's not something I usually talk about. Too many friends have avoided me after they found out, scared to be associated with my family. I didn't want that to happen with you," he confesses. "Besides, most people never know. I'm nothing like my dad. I don't look like him, and I don't act like him."

Pity stirs in me, as I think of the people who have rejected Stewart based only on his last name. Guilt follows. How am I any better? I'm using Stewart for his last name at this very second.

I spot Rafe and Shelly with their heads close together, whispering in the hallway that leads to the office and the safe. I glance away, fearful Stewart will follow my gaze and recognize my friends. Shelly disappears, while Rafe takes up his position as a look-out, using his newly bulked-up body to block the hallway entrance.

"It's true," I agree. "You don't favor your dad." Johnny's face is all sharp angles, while Stewart's is softer.

I try to focus on his response, but it's a struggle to not constantly check the clock resting on the fireplace mantle to my right, which reads a quarter past midnight. We had timed this all out. How long it should take Shelly to get into the office and turn off the cameras, using Stewart's keycard. How long to enter a set of numbers that Rafe had mysteriously obtained into the safe's numeric keypad. How long to put the valuables into the black duffle bag Shelly brought and then for Shelly and Rafe to escape using the stairs next to the elevator. The clock hands turn with maddening slowness.

Stewart grimaces, continuing our conversation. "My dad wanted a sporty, aggressive kid, but instead he got me—nerdy and shy." He sighs, swirling the champagne in his glass.

Guilt bites me even harder, digging in. I'm about to respond when the same security guard with the earpiece appears at Stewart's shoulder. He talks softly to Stewart, who frowns and listens intently. I'm convinced the guard is telling him about Shelly and the safe. Any minute now, alarms will sound and the guards will grab me. I hold my breath, muscles tense.

After the man leaves, Stewart tells me, "I'm sorry for the interruption, but I need to talk to my dad and then I have to do a few things in his office. I'll be gone 20 minutes tops. Is that okay?"

My heart slams loudly against my ribs. All I can hear is the word *office*. The room where Shelly is right now. Stewart can't go there.

Forcing a smile I say, "Of course. No problem."

As I watch him walk toward Johnny, my thoughts spin. What can I do to stall him until Shelly finishes with the safe? Panic makes my mind go blank.

Rafe's normal look of studied indifference slips when he sees me walking his way, replaced by alarm. This isn't what we discussed. I'm supposed to ignore Rafe and Shelly. To walk out of this evening on Stewart's arm—the perfect alibi. Now that plan is blown, but what am I supposed to do? Let Stewart catch Shelly? Watch the police drag her away? No way. I've battled for her before, and I'll do it again. After all, she's family to me.

I come to a halt, standing a few feet away from the hallway that leads to the office. "Stewart's coming here in a minute," I hiss at Rafe under my breath as I stare through the crowd, fixated on Stewart. Judging by body language, he's almost done talking to his dad.

I whisper more desperately, "Rafe!"

His eyes roam the room, looking for a solution.

Stewart leaves Johnny and makes his way toward us. Thankfully, he's preoccupied, looking down at his phone as he walks.

"What're we going to do?" My voice is tight with anxiety.

"Distract him and buy Shelly more time," Rafe says decisively. He jolts into motion like a man waking from a dream. For the second time this evening, he grabs my arm and drags me along, heading for the dance floor.

"Distract him? How?" My voice rises in panic as I watch Stewart approach.

Rafe halts on the edge of the dance floor and pulls me to him. "Easy. Jealousy." With that, he draws me close and begins to sway. The song is a slow one, with an underlying sensuous beat. He moves like liquid mercury, with fluid limbs and glinting eyes. I hadn't been lying when I told Stewart I'm not a good dancer, but it doesn't seem to matter with Rafe. His grip on me is firm, and all I do is follow his rhythm.

He brushes his hands down to my waist, pulling our lower bodies flush. His hips roll in time to the music, brushing against me in a rhythmic pattern. Desire rises, scalding through me at his touch. Rafe stares down at me with a dark intensity that makes me press closer, wanting more of him. His fingers tighten, digging into the tender flesh just above my hip bones. My arms wrap tight around his neck, and I push up into him. I tilt my head up, imagining what it would be like to kiss him, right in front of everyone. The rest of the room and the fear about my mom and this robbery all fade until I only focus on the points of my body that are in contact with his.

Rafe gazes intimately into my eyes. "Is he looking?"

"What?" I ask dreamily.

More impatient now, Rafe says, "Is he watching us? Is it working?"

As if a bucket of cold water has been poured over my head, I snap back into the here and now. "Oh." I peer over Rafe's shoulder, searching for Stewart. He's standing at the entrance to the hallway leading to the office, staring at me with obvious confusion and pain.

Guiltily, I try to push away from Rafe, to put some space between us, but he holds me tight.

"He's by the hallway entrance," I tell Rafe, my head dropping with embarrassment. Stewart had seen it all. He had seen the way I looked at Rafe, the way our bodies moved together. I had told him I didn't want to dance but here I was, brazen on the dance floor with another man. Even though it's necessary to protect Shelly, the burn of shame is hot on my cheeks.

54

An angry voice rings out, rising above the sound of the music. At first, I ignore it, too full of guilt over Stewart. But the argument gains in volume until it's impossible to disregard. Dancing couples next to me halt their movement and turn to find the source. Rafe and I do the same. My champagne glass sits on a side table where I had placed it. I pick it up and drink. There's an urge in me to keep on drinking until I wash away the memory of Stewart's expression as he watched me dance with Rafe.

Rafe turns to see what the commotion is all about, and I follow his gaze. Johnny the Shark is quarreling with an older, gray-haired man across the room. The man's face is crimson with anger. Johnny has his hand up, palm facing the man like he's trying to calm him down.

With horror, I stare as the man draws a small pistol from inside his jacket. He aims it at Johnny's chest and shoots him point blank. The bullet must go through Johnny's body because a second later the enormous window behind him shatters with a deafening crash. The sound is so loud that I flinch, spilling champagne across the bodice of my mom's white dress. Shards of glass rain down both inside and outside the room.

For a minute, everything goes eerily still. The DJ, the clinking of glasses, the roar of conversation—it all ceases. Then chaos breaks loose. Someone in the crowd screams, high and shrieking. People start running, and I lose track of the gunman. Most of the guests sprint toward the exit, but some move toward Johnny, who, with a shocked expression, slumps to the ground. Stewart passes me without a word, heading to his father.

I stand frozen, staring at the empty window frame with jagged pieces of glass lining its edges. When someone touches my arm, I wheel around with my hand raised to strike. It's Shelly, who recoils at the sight of my upraised fist. Rafe grabs my hand before I can lash out and gently returns it to my side.

"Tiffany," says Shelly, speaking slowly like she's talking to a small child. "It's me. We need to get out of here." She holds up a worn black duffle bag, bulging unevenly from the contents within it.

I must be in shock from just having witnessed a man get shot, because I stare at the bag dumbly, unclear for a second why it's important. Then it dawns on me. It worked. Shelly got into the safe. We got the money.

I can help my mom.

"Go!" Rafe urges us, and we do, rushing toward the exit. I spare a last look at Johnny. I can't see him. There are too many onlookers. In the shifting crowd, I get a glimpse of Stewart, clutching an earpiece and shouting into it.

Rafe slams open the door leading into the hallway with the mirrored ceiling and marble floor. Pushing through the frightened throng of guests into the hall, we rush to the door for the stairs. Praying that it won't set off an alarm, I push the door open. No bells ring. No sirens wail.

The three of us dash down the stairs, going round and round in an ever-descending spiral. I concentrate on not falling. The high heels I'm wearing make me slower than my companions.

Guests from the masquerade ball stream into the stairwell behind us. Their panicked voices follow us as they escape the chaos of the overcrowded hallway. Their footsteps ring on the concrete steps. The quicker people flow around me and pass, heading downstairs. I'm hoping that with all these people we'll be lost in the shuffle. Just another set of guests running from the shooting, rather than criminals fleeing from a robbery.

We descend for what seems like forever, then at a sign that reads 40th we exit onto a floor filled with hotel rooms. There's a long central hallway and doors lining the walls on each side. The room numbers scroll by in my periphery as we run: 4220, 4218, 4216.

I keep expecting to hear the sound of pursuit behind us, but so far there's only silence. Maybe everyone is too distracted by the shooting to worry about us. I hope that's the case.

At the end of the hallway is a bank of six elevators for the general hotel guests. A group of young women wait by the elevator doors. They're all dressed in similar tight short skirts with matching tube tops. In their center is a woman with a revealing white dress. A sash around her chest reads, "bride to be." The women lean against each other, slurring their words and talking with overly loud voices.

Shelly, Rafe, and I press in close to the group, trying to blend in with them. The elevator chimes, and we all crowd in together. This is one of the riskiest parts of our plan. If someone discovers the empty safe, the police could already be on the ground floor, waiting for us to step off the elevator and right into custody.

The descent stops, and noiselessly the elevator doors slide open to reveal the lobby. There's no security waiting for us. It's a clear path to the main doors of the hotel. Walking fast but trying not to run, we head for the exit.

We almost make it, are close enough to feel the incoming rush of fresh air, when I hear it. The ringing of the phone on the security desk. We'll have to pass right by it. In slow motion, I watch the guard pick up the phone and talk into the receiver. He looks up and scans the crowd until his eyes fall on us. They light in recognition.

"Run!" shouts Rafe, and he takes off, sprinting to the door. Shelly is right behind him. Stumbling in my stupid high heels, I run after. The security guard comes around his desk, almost reaching me, when I push through to the outside. The blare of taxicabs angrily honking sounds like the sweet music of freedom.

Rafe and Shelly have pulled ahead, half a block in front of me. I pause to kick off my shoes into the bushes. The guard has also made it through the main entrance and is outside on the sidewalk. I ignore his shout of "Stop!" and run faster than I've ever done in my entire life.

Startled tourists stare at me with wide eyes when I rush past. The soles of my bare feet sting as they slap the pavement. After a few blocks, Rafe turns off a side street in front of me. Three blocks later, Shelly disappears into a Chinese restaurant.

Sirens break out behind me, their warbling cry getting closer as I hurtle down the Strip. I take a sharp right and dash into the first casino I see. A police car with flashing lights passes as I watch, half-hidden in the shadows, peeking through the window. It is headed toward the Luxor. When I pull back from the window, it acts as a mirror, reflecting my wide horrified eyes and the mask that still obscures half my face. I had forgotten it was on. With revulsion, I rip it off and stuff it into my pocket. I don't ever want to see it again. It's the embodiment of my shame, my subterfuge.

In the hotel gift shop, I buy a baggy hoodie sweatshirt with the words Las Vegas spelled out in gaudy rhinestones and matching sweatpants. My mom's white dress is stained from the spilled champagne. Ruined. Regretfully, I throw the dress away, shoving it down deep in the women's bathroom trash can and piling crumpled paper towels on top.

In my new clothing, I step back out onto the brightly lit Strip. People around me laugh and talk. They smile and embrace. In my distressed state, their faces appear distorted, like in a carnival fun house. Everything is upside down, and that's when I realize I've been lying to myself. I thought I could do these things, bad things, and when they were done I'd go back to my normal life. Now I see so clearly that after tonight nothing will ever be the same.

55

We meet up at the Starlight, like we planned, in the back of the decaying hotel. Once this space had held an upscale steakhouse. Only torn and dusty leather booths remain. Rafe, Shelly, and I avoid them, instead standing in a loose semicircle in the center of the room.

Now that I've stopped running, the enormity of my actions, the reality of my situation, hits me. It's a blow to my head, to my heart. I can't believe I did those awful, terrible things. I betrayed Stewart, committed a crime, and watched a man get shot. It's all too much. I'm shaking. My body trembles like a leaf in the wind. Tears well in my eyes and tumble down my cheeks.

"Wh—what just happened?" I ask Rafe and Shelly, crying. "What did we do? I'm so confused. Who shot Johnny?"

"Who knows?" Rafe shrugs, unmoved. "I've never seen that guy before."

"Are you saying you had nothing to do with it?" I cry, fearful that I'm an accomplice to a murder. Worried that I'm going to jail, rather than to college. How could I have been so stupid? To let Rafe and Shelly drag me into this mess. But I can't blame them, not if I'm being honest. They may have pointed out this road, but I'm the one who walked down it.

"Me?" Rafe barks out a harsh laugh. "Trust me, I don't have that kind of clout. I'm small-time compared to those guys."

Can I trust him? Everything's changed since I saw Stewart's father get shot. My attention turns to Shelly to see how she's handling everything. It startles me that she has the same look as Rafe. That determined, flat expression, like nothing that's occurred can touch her. Like she's buried in a block of ice.

"How can you be so calm right now?" I ask them both. "We just saw a man get shot. He's probably dead. He—" My voice rises, along with my panic.

"Tiffany," Rafe says, cutting me off, "there's nothing we can do about that. It's out of our control. We need to hurry, finish our business." He turns to Shelly, gesturing to the now-dirty duffle bag by her feet. "Let's see it."

Kneeling, she unzips the bag and opens it wide. Even through my tears, I gasp at the stacks of bills, coins, casino chips, and sparkling jewels resting there. Rafe lets out a long whistle and selects a single $1,000 casino chip. He flips it up in the air and catches it in his palm. "Give Tiffany her share," he tells Shelly.

After a brief search through the bag, Shelly pulls out a stack of bills bound together with a thin strip of paper. She passes it over to me. I take it with unsteady hands, staring at the thick wad of money. When I hear the sound of a zipper, I glance up to see Shelly closing the bag. It's still full. Shelly has moved over to stand by Rafe, on the opposite side of the circle from me. Clutching the bag to her chest, she refuses to meet my eyes.

Dread lodges in my throat. I attempt to swallow it down. "Guys?" I sniffle. "What's going on?"

Rafe lifts his chin. "That's it. Your cut of the money."

Shocked, I rock back like they slapped me. "B—but we said we would split it evenly. This is only a few thousand dollars. It's not enough to cover my mom's treatments." Shaking the stack of money at them, I take a deep breath, trying to calm my racing heart.

Something isn't right here.

"We talked about it and decided that's what you get," says Rafe flatly.

"We? Shelly?" I try to capture my best friend's gaze.

When she finally looks up, her jaw is tight and her eyes are cold. "Rafe's right, Tiffany. We did most of the dangerous work, so it's only fair we get the bulk of it. Besides, we need to buy plane tickets."

"What are you talking about?" I'm reeling, a pit of dread spreading through my chest.

She shifts the bag up to her shoulder and confirms my worst fear. "We're leaving."

Astonished, I watch Shelly wrap her hand around Rafe's biceps and lean into him. It's a declaration of possession, like he belongs to her, like she's claiming him. I look at Rafe, trying to figure out what I'm seeing, to make sense of it. A flicker of dark emotion rushes across his face. Regret? Sorrow? Anger?

"I warned you to stay away from us." Rafe's voice is toneless, his expression grim.

Stunned, I clutch the money to my chest. "I don't understand."

A cruel smile from Shelly, and it all becomes clear. The roller coaster is over. I'm being unceremoniously pushed off the ride so it can go on without me. I can't believe that Shelly, of all people, would do this to me. It's killing me, seeing them touch each other, the familiarity in that gesture. All the dreams I had about Rafe, how I would be his savior. Instead, he and Shelly have damned me.

How they must have laughed at me behind my back. Silly little Tiffany and her schoolgirl crush. So naïve. So easy to manipulate. "You set me up, and now you're leaving? With the police after me? Probably the Mafia, too." My voice breaks. Tears fill my throat, choking me. Rafe's dishonesty stings, a shallow cut. Shelly's betrayal is a death blow, a knife straight through my back and into my heart.

I won't *ever* love again. This hurts too badly.

"You knew exactly what you were doing," Shelly spits out, angry at me for reasons I don't fully understand.

As I absorb this new reality, I realize that Shelly is leaving. Rafe is leaving. My mother is dying.

I'll be alone.

This is a nightmare. Every bad dream coming true at once. "Shelly," I plead raggedly, "please, you can't leave me."

Eyes like flint with no spark, she says dully, "I have to go. There's nothing for me here."

"*I'm* here." There's a void opening in me, vast and empty.

"Yeah, for how long? How long until you go off to college, Tiffany? How long until *you* are the one that leaves *me*? If I don't go now, I'll be stuck here forever. I'll end up just like my mom." Shelly's detached façade breaks, and her voice becomes raw. Her eyes glisten with tears to match the ones that spill unbidden down my cheeks.

That stops me. There's truth to her words. I've known for a long time that we're on different paths. We have never envisioned the same future, not even when we were young.

"Let me go, Tiffany. I have to go." She softens even more, begging. Her tears overflow and run freely.

But how can I do that? Let her go when she's all I'll have left? I can't. I'm not strong enough.

"Please," she whispers, needing my mercy, my forgiveness, my permission.

I love her, and I hate her.

I nod once, sobbing.

There's nothing left to be said. Rafe pulls the heavy duffle from Shelly, slinging it over his shoulder. Without a good-bye, they hold hands and walk away. No longer able to stand, I crumple to my knees and watch through tear-streaked eyes until the darkness swallows them.

I desperately gasp for breath, my chest a gaping, painful wound.

If heartbreak can kill you, then I'm going to die.

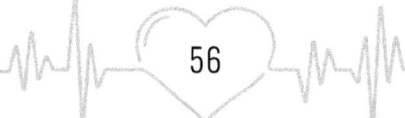

56

It's not me who dies.

It's my mother.

One month after Shelly and Rafe leave, she loses her battle with cancer. Her rose-covered casket goes into the ground and, with it, my heart.

57

"You have to eat, my dear." Mr. Chen leaves the steamed dumplings, my favorite, on the nightstand. It sits there, next to an ever-growing pile of dirty dishes with barely-picked-at food and half-drunk drinks.

I've fallen apart. Broken into pieces like a plate thrown at a wall. Spending as much time as I can in bed, I stare up at the ceiling fan as it spins lazily over my head. I'm getting bad grades, ruining my chance to be valedictorian and any hope of being accepted into an Ivy League college. Those dreams have blown away like dandelion seeds on the wind.

I can't even bother to be upset by it. Everything feels distant. My life is a dream that someone else is having—or, more likely, a nightmare. Idly, I wonder if the police are ever going to come to arrest me. I almost hope they do. My guilt over Stewart and how I used him demands payment. If I go to jail, it will all be so simple. No more worrying about school or looking over my shoulder waiting for the handcuffs.

But no flashing sirens pull into the apartment parking lot. No one comes for me. How did I get away with it? Surely they have discovered the empty safe by now? The only answer seems the least probable, that someone covered for me. The person with that kind of access and power is Stewart, but he wouldn't protect me after the way I'd treated him. Would he?

I've kept an eye on the newspapers, waiting to see my name in the headlines. There's been no mention of the robbery. The death of Johnny the Shark has been widely reported on, however. His killer, the older man I saw, died in a shoot-out with the police when he tried to escape the penthouse. I imagine that long hallway with mirrors in the ceiling and the marble floor covered in blood.

Apparently, the murderer was a leading member of a rival mob. The newspapers report that the fight was over disputed territory in New York, where the gangs and mobsters each wanted their own piece of the drug trade.

"Tiffany, eat," Mr. Chen chides again.

I don't bother to answer. Pulling the covers over my head, I roll away from him and shut out the world.

ENEMIES AND LOVERS

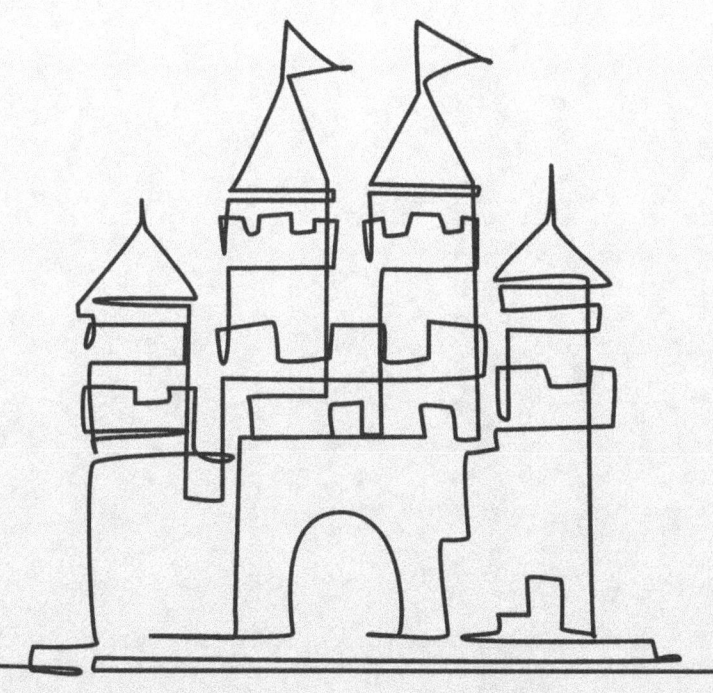

PRESENT, ORLANDO, FLORIDA

The conference is boring. With the lights down low and considering how tired I am from yesterday, it's a struggle to stay awake. I'm into my third cup of coffee but can't stop yawning. The only thing keeping me from falling into a complete stupor is Ethan's presence beside me. Sneakily glancing at him in the dark, with only the glow from the presenter's screen at the front of the room, I trace the lines of his face as my daydreaming mind wanders. Those straight eyebrows, the tiny scar. That cleft chin and stubble-covered jaw. That full bottom lip. What would he taste like? How would he feel? My gaze travels to his powerful arms and broad chest, remembering how solid he was sleeping next to me last night. Large hands with ropy veins along the back.

Without looking over, Ethan writes on a napkin and slides it across to me. *Why are you staring at me like I'm candy and you're a kid on Halloween?*

With an embarrassed intake of breath, I rip my eyes off him and whip my body to face forward. In my peripheral vision, I see his shoulders shaking with suppressed laughter. Annoyed that he called me out, I scoot my chair a few inches away with a disgruntled *hmph*. I cross my arms over my chest and glare ahead, tuning into the lecture on inhalational lung disease.

Ethan's laughter becomes louder, and a few heads glance our way. "Don't be like that, Tiffy," he whispers and reaches out to grab hold of my chair. With one quick tug, he easily pulls me back over to him. Now we're sitting even closer, our shoulders almost touching. Ethan snatches the napkin and flips it over to the blank side. He bends his head over it, scribbling furiously. Curiosity makes me crane my head around, trying to see what he's doing.

He finishes writing and slides the note across the table like a blackjack dealer.

I'm bored. When can we leave?

I take the pen from his hand and write back.

The lectures are done at three.

Ethan pulls the pen from my hand almost before I'm finished writing.

I'm not going to make it. Let's get out of here.

I take the pen, noting how warm it is from Ethan's fingers.

We can't. I don't want to get in trouble.

Ethan snorts derisively when he reads my response.

How could you get in trouble? No one knows us here. Who's going to tell? I want to go to Epcot early!

Good point. Everyone here is focused on the presentation. Who would notice if we left?

Ethan's already shoving his papers into his bag when I write back.

Okay. Let's go.

Giggling like school kids, we burst out of the hotel lobby doors and into an overcast Orlando day. Fluffy gray clouds drift and swirl overhead. It's dry for now, but the air smells metallic. A rainstorm is coming.

"Look," says Ethan, pointing, "there's a bus about to leave for Epcot. Let's catch it."

A large red bus with a huge Mickey Mouse face plastered on its side sits idling in the roundabout in front of our hotel. It looks like it just arrived, with a long line of passengers waiting to enter.

Ethan starts toward the bus.

"Wait." I place my hand on his chest, stopping him. "Should we go upstairs and change first?"

"And miss the bus? Who knows how long we'd have to wait for the next one? Let's go now." He's all anxious excitement, a kid on Christmas morning.

"But I'm wearing a skirt." I gesture at my body.

A suggestive grin spreads across Ethan's face. "And you're wearing it quite well, if you don't mind me saying." He pretends to lean around and stare at my backside. Apparently, he still has a thing for sexy librarians.

"Ethan!" I swat his arm, laughing.

"Do you need to go back? I guess you should change your shoes." He glances at my sensible low heels, a frown of concern wiping away his crooked smile.

"No, it's fine. These shoes are surprisingly comfortable," I tell him honestly.

The last of the line of people is boarding the bus.

"Great. Let's go." Ethan holds out his hand. I take it and together we run to catch the bus. We get there right before the driver closes the door. He lets us in with a disgruntled stare.

Squeezing past standing bodies and baby strollers, we move to the back. At the next stop, most of the people exit, so we sit down. I push my fingers through my hair, separating it strand by strand. The damp Florida humidity makes it curl. "I feel so naughty. I can't believe we just skipped out on the rest of the lectures like that."

Ethan quirks an eyebrow at me. "What? You never did that before? Skipped out on classes, back in high school and college, to go have some fun? Didn't you ever lie to your mom and sneak out of the house?"

Shaking my head, I answer, "When my mom was sick and right after she died, I missed a lot of school, but I never ditched for fun."

I don't tell him about how I may not have ditched school, but I definitely have snuck around. All those nights of lying to my mom and Mr. Chen when I went to the Strip. How would Ethan react if I mentioned that? Would he push me away with revulsion? Reject me? I can't keep him in the dark forever, but the thought of losing his respect and trust is too painful.

Chuckling, he says, "Well, we're going to have to change that. Priority number one is making sure Tiffy has the best day ever so she won't feel guilty about missing the lectures."

His arm lays draped along the back of my seat. When I shift back, Ethan doesn't move. Instead, he curls his fingers so they gently brush the top of my shoulder. Just a casual touch, so small, and yet my breath catches at the sensation.

The bus rumbles along the street. I angle my body toward him. "I like that plan. It can't be *too* much fun though. Otherwise, I might just skip the rest of this conference."

"Now you're giving me a challenge," teases Ethan.

"Uh-oh." I laugh. "You're going to ruin me, aren't you?"

"I certainly hope so." Ethan's giving me that dark sexy look again and the way he says it, like it's a promise for later, sends a tingle deep into my lower stomach.

The bus jolts to a stop, and it's time to get out. After we scan through the gates, I lead us deeper into the park. Ethan's silent at my side as we walk. There's a thoughtful, almost sad expression on his face. Eventually, he says, "I'm sorry your mom passed away. I was thinking about how difficult that must've been for you."

Ah, that's what has been making him so unusually quiet.

"How old were you when that happened, if you don't mind me asking?" he says softly.

I wait for the depressed feeling I often get when I think back to that time, but it doesn't happen. I'm calm, like maybe I can have this conversation and come out on the other side and still be okay. It's a new thought that grief doesn't have to be my only companion.

"I had just turned 18." I lift my gaze to his, taking comfort in his now-familiar features.

The line between his eyebrows deepens. "Who took care of you? I think you said you don't really have family."

"A neighbor, Mr. Chen, who was close to my mother and me, took me in. He was like family to us. Legally, I was an adult and didn't need a guardian, but emotionally I was a wreck. He watched over me. If I hadn't had him… well, I don't want to think of what would have happened."

I let out a deep sigh. "Mr. Chen was great, but he was old. He got really sick less than a year after losing my mom. That was a turning point for me. I had stopped caring about anything by then. Didn't care about school or my future anymore. Mr. Chen made me promise to try again. He had been a doctor in Taiwan. Right before he died, I swore I would continue his legacy and go to medical school."

I remember it, first one coffin going into the ground, then eight months later another coffin, another funeral. More sadness that made me feel like I was there with them, buried six feet deep. Like I'd never see the light again.

Ethan stops walking and stares at me, his face filled with quiet sympathy. "How did you survive it? I hate how you had to go through that, especially alone. If I had known you back then, I could have helped."

Right there, in the middle of the walkway, with people flowing around us like water parting for two boulders, Ethan pulls me roughly to his chest. He hugs me tight. At first, my hands hang at my sides. I'm overwhelmed by his close proximity and by memories from my past. How different things could have been for me if I had known Ethan back then. How things could have been better if Shelly had stayed by my side. But Shelly had abandoned me. I'm worried that eventually everyone else, including Ethan, will leave me too.

This realization hits hard. I've spent the past decade of my life pushing everyone away, so I wouldn't have to experience that kind of pain again. With tears pricking the backs of my eyes, my hands come alive and wrap around him, returning the hug.

Muffled against his firm chest, I murmur, "I wish I had known you back then, too."

He pulls away and looks at me tenderly while I swallow my tears. Even though I'm working hard to let Ethan in, I still don't like to cry in front of him.

"Man, I'm not doing a very good job of giving Tiffany the most fun day of her life so far, am I?" He frowns. "I ask you about sad stuff and dredge up memories you might not want to face."

"It's okay." Seeing his doubtful expression, I repeat. "*Really*, it's okay. I'm glad you asked. Most people don't know what to say when someone you love dies so they stay silent, but that doesn't help. I'm glad we talked."

"Then I'm glad too."

T he Test Track ride leaves my hair tangled and my eyes stinging. It was fast and jarring, and I loved it. "What did you think?" I ask Ethan as we walk off the ride. I'm practically skipping, so invigorated by the experience.

"It was awesome. I can't believe those cars go 60 miles per hour." Ethan looks around as the walkway splits in three directions in front of us. Not sure which way to go, he asks, "What's next?"

I consult my mental map. Epcot has two main sections—a front section that is mostly rides and a back section called the World Showcase. The World Showcase surrounds a large lake and has 11 different pavilions that each feature a different country. The architecture of each pavilion matches its country, and in each one there's native food and shopping. I suggest we go there. Ethan nods in agreement.

We walk through the first couple of countries, stopping to window shop and people watch. When we get to the Germany pavilion, Ethan asks to get lunch. It's getting late, so I agree. A quick-service restaurant advertises authentic bratwurst. The spicy sausage is delicious, on a fresh-baked bun with house-made chips.

Not wanting to take the time to sit down and eat, we munch as we walk. There's a chill in the late fall air. Dry leaves and a few stray pieces of dropped popcorn skitter by our feet, stirred by the breeze. A shiver runs through me as a particularly strong gust sends my hair flying.

Without a word, Ethan takes off his coat and places it over my shoulders.

The jacket is still warm from his body. I shove my arms into the sleeves, liking how they're too long and hang over my hands, keeping my fingers toasty. Hoping Ethan won't notice, I turn my nose to the collar and inhale his clean scent. It's comforting, the now familiar blend of soap, laundry, and mint. I settle deeper into the jacket with a contented sigh.

Ethan's watching me, a tiny smile lighting up his face. "You're different now from how you were when I first met you. It's like you're lighter, sunnier. Like you've bloomed."

I think about how he's right and wonder if he realizes how much he has to do with my transformation. It's from spending time with him that I'm learning to trust and be happy again. I want to grab that joy and keep it with me, but what if I'm not always able to hold onto it? Would he reject me then? Leave me like I've been left before?

"Do you like me better this way?" I ask tentatively.

Without hesitation, he answers, "I like you *all* ways, happy and sad. I like all the Tiffany's past, present, and future. I'll take them all."

His words turn a key deep in my heart, opening doors that have been locked for far too long.

A kiosk on the edge of the Italian pavilion catches Ethan's attention. It's a small brown building with a tile roof. A sign on the side advertises gelato and cannoli.

Ethan eyes it hungrily. "Should we stop?"

"*Really*? You're still hungry? We just had lunch." I shake my head, amazed at the capacity of his stomach.

He grins crookedly. "Don't you know that there are two stomachs, Tiffy? One for regular food and another for dessert?"

I'm trying, and failing, to suppress my smile. "Hmm…weird. I don't remember learning that in anatomy class."

"It's a fact. Just ask any eight-year-old." Ethan angles off toward the gelato shop, walking quickly.

"You're admitting to your immaturity? Identifying with eight-year-olds." I follow him into the line of people waiting for the icy Italian treats.

"I admit to nothing," he says, smirking.

We read the menu, debating about what we should get. I tell him, "My mom used to make home-made cannoli. It was delicious. Totally spoiled me. I don't even bother trying it anywhere else. Nothing will be as good as hers."

"That sounds amazing," says Ethan. In unison, we step forward in the line. "Was she a good cook?"

"The best. Made pasta from scratch. Cooked her own marinara. I don't know where she learned it, but Italian was her favorite." It comes back to me, the bubbling pot on the stove. The smell of oregano and sauteed tomatoes. How that aroma would fill our entire apartment and waft down the stairs. Shelly would inevitably knock on our door when she smelled it, on the hunt for a rare home-cooked meal.

We reach the front of the line, and I get a single scoop of vanilla, which earns me an eye roll from Ethan and some mumbling about how my taste buds are "boring." He chooses the Coppa Amarena, a concoction of vanilla and cherry gelato topped with amaretto cookies, whipped cream, and chocolate shavings. Even I admit it looks delicious.

We carry our gelato over an arching bridge to a small pier that juts out into the lake. Colorful striped poles rise out of the water. An authentic-looking black-lacquered Venetian gondola is docked before us. It's just like pictures of Italy that I've seen in books and magazines.

Ethan and I sit on a bench with our backs to the main walkway. He stretches his legs out, rubs his right knee, and then crosses his ankles.

"You okay with all this walking?" I slowly lick the sweet vanilla gelato off the back of my spoon.

"It's fine." He lets out a contented sigh and leans back, slanting his face up to the sky as the breeze teases his hair, ruffling it like a lover's fingers.

It's peaceful where we sit, surrounded by the lake on three sides. Small wavelets stirred by the wind ripple across the blue-gray surface. A snowy white bird with a curved beak, an ibis I think, comes to perch on the metal railing. Ethan tosses up a piece of his cookie, which the bird catches in midair. With a whoosh of wings, it takes off to enjoy the snack.

Storm clouds slowly gather overhead. The wind has picked up, and even in Ethan's jacket I shiver. He notices and slides closer. He hesitates, then puts his arm around me and pulls me tight against his side.

We keep ending up like this, I think, touching one another. It's like we're magnets getting pulled together over and over. I allow my head to lean back on Ethan's warm shoulder. He shifts into a more comfortable position as I ease myself against him.

"This feels nice," I tell him. It's a dangerous thing to say. To admit that all this looking and touching hasn't been by accident.

"It does," Ethan murmurs against my hair, sending a shiver through my body that has nothing to do with the cold. "*You* feel nice." His breath is hot across my scalp. His hand rubs up and down my arm, chaffing it, trying to warm me.

"You too," I whisper back, glad he can't see my face right now. My stomach tightens, and there's a tingling growing deep within my belly. It's absurd. If this little bit of contact gives me butterflies, what would it be like to kiss him?

I lift my head from his shoulder to find him staring into my eyes. We're inches apart. Ethan watches intently as I push closer, rising slightly off the bench to meet his height. I close the distance between us. He holds absolutely still, like he's afraid to break a spell.

I kiss him.

It's a soft kiss, gentle and yielding. Ethan's lips are silken, and his mouth is sweet from the gelato. I sense he's holding back, letting me take the lead like he doesn't want to scare me off.

I'm not scared, though. I'm awash with desire. It burns through any remaining trepidation, leaving my insecurities in ashes. More confident now, I kiss him harder. His mouth falls open with a sigh, and I sweep my tongue in to meet his.

The contact is electric, a shot of adrenaline straight to my core. I wrap my arms tightly around the back of his neck and turn to him fully, getting as close as I can.

Ethan's restraint slips. His hands rise to tangle in my hair, fingers kneading the tender skin behind my ear and at the base of my head. Then his right hand runs lightly down along my jaw. He takes my chin and lifts it, angling my mouth to deepen our kiss. It's so delicious that a soft moan escapes my parted lips. The sound of it wakes me out of the desire-induced stupor I've slipped into.

"Oh." I pull away, my hand coming up to touch my kiss-swollen lips. Wide-eyed, I stare at Ethan, who looks back cautiously. When I let out a low laugh and drop my hand to settle on his shoulder, a relieved smile spreads across his face. He must have been worried about my reaction.

Blinking, I take a couple of slow breaths of air. I'm trying to get my heart rate under control, to marshal the desire that still dominates my body. "Sorry," I say and shake my head ruefully. "I didn't mean to make out with you in the middle of Disney World."

Ethan lets out a shaky laugh. "Trust me, Tiffy, you have no reason to apologize. You can kiss me anywhere, anytime."

He's having a hard time catching his breath as well, I note with some satisfaction. At least I wasn't the only one stirred up.

"Especially if you kiss me like that," he adds.

Trying to harness my newly rediscovered inner flirt, I gaze up at him through my eyelashes. "Are you implying that I'm going to kiss you again, Ethan Clark?"

"I hope so," he answers. We sit there like idiots, grinning at each other as if we've discovered the cure for all the world's unhappiness.

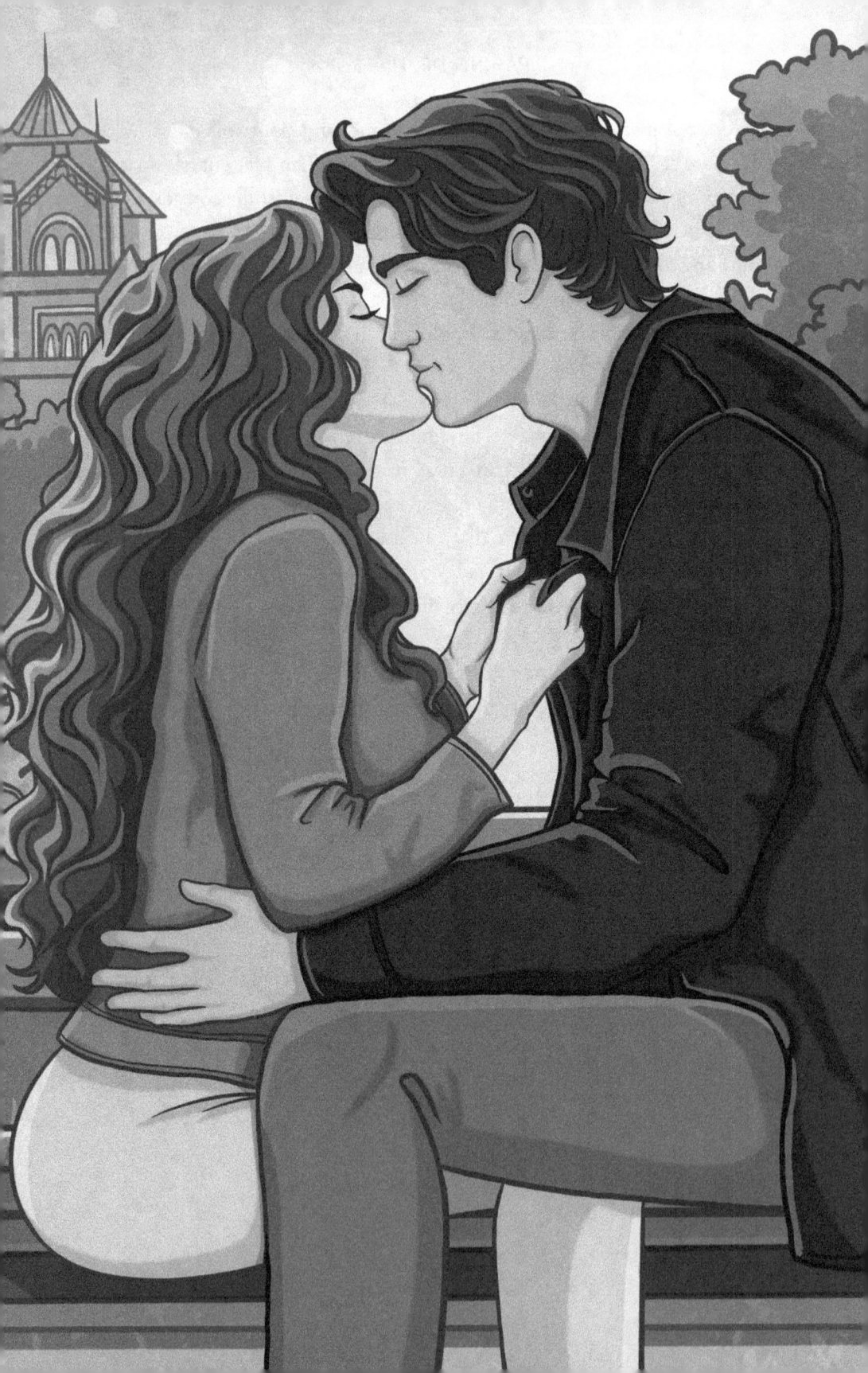

60

After snuggling for a little longer, Ethan straightens. "Hate to ruin the moment, but I need to use the restroom."

"Me too," I admit, my breathing slowly returning to normal.

We throw away the remainder of our now-melted gelato. The men's and women's restrooms are on opposite ends of the square, so we agree to meet back in front of the bell tower.

My mind is scattered, so busy reliving the kiss that I walk right past the entrance to the women's bathroom not just once, but twice. I admonish myself to concentrate and finally make it in. Once I'm done and back outside, I search for Ethan, but he's not at our designated meet-up spot yet. My phone vibrates.

> *Melanie: Hey. Can I buy Fred some treats?*
>
> *Tiffany: Just got a brand-new box. Out already?*
>
> *Melanie: Used them all. What can I say? Fred has me wrapped around his paw. So cute when he begs.*
>
> *Tiffany: Lol. Okay. Get more treats. Wow. You're turning into a cat person.*
>
> *Melanie: I know! OK, serious question.*
>
> *Tiffany: ???*

Melanie: When U get back, will U come to the shelter with me? I want to adopt a kitty!!

Tiffany: Really? Of course, I'll go.

Melanie: It'll be so fun. We can have cat play dates and take them on walks together.

Tiffany: Ummm…not how cats work. You're thinking of dogs.

Melanie: Ohhh. Explains a lot. Yesterday, I took Fred on a walk, and he just laid there. Had to drag him along the sidewalk. Wondered if he was tired or something? Everyone kept giving me weird looks.

Tiffany: What???

Melanie: So anyway, how's Mickey Mouse?

Tiffany: Amazing. The best!

Melanie: Ethan have anything to do with that?

Tiffany: Well…

Melanie: NO WAY! What happened? Spill it.

Tiffany: We kinda kissed.

Melanie: OMG! I knew it! Knew it from that first day. At UR wedding, I want all the credit.

Tiffany: Slow down the crazy train. It was one kiss.

Melanie: There'll be more, right?

Tiffany: Hope so.

Tiffany: Keep it between us. Might not work out.

Melanie: Give him a chance, okay? Don't sabotage it.

Tiffany: Okay.

Melanie: I have a good feeling about this.

Tiffany: Can't believe I'm saying this, but I do too.

Melanie: When you get home, I want ALL the details. Promise?

Tiffany: Promise.

I'm grinning at my phone, thinking about how funny Melanie is when I notice the large work boots that have entered my field of vision. They walk right up to me. I lift my gaze and look straight into a pair of cat-green eyes.

My breath catches in my throat.

No.

It can't be?

Can it?

Sure enough, the man standing in front of me is Rafe, all grown up. He's the same, but different. Sleeves of tattoos so dark I can't make out the individual images crawl up arms thick with corded muscle. Another tattoo licks up the side of his neck, ending below his ear. He's gotten taller, at least another foot since I last saw him. Broader and filled out with bulging muscles everywhere. Dark stubble covers his jaw and arches over an unsmiling mouth. His hair is black as midnight, wavy, and long enough to curl against the collar of his shirt.

He's beautiful in a brutal kind of way.

The worst feature, the thing that I can't look away from, are his eyes. They glitter, cold and merciless.

As I stand frozen, my mind spinning from shock, Rafe silently reaches his hand toward my chest. For a moment, I think he's going to hurt me, maybe push me, but instead he picks up the conference badge that dangles from its long red lanyard against my sternum. The one I had forgotten I was wearing. He lifts it up to read, eyes narrowing.

Minutes ago, with Ethan, I had felt like I was floating. Now, staring at Rafe, I'm free falling, plummeting to the ground from a great height. My stomach turns, nausea rising up my throat. There's a roaring in my ears, the sound of the ocean during a storm. It's so loud that I almost don't hear Ethan call my name.

"Tiffany." Ethan's voice is a thunderclap, waking me up from this nightmare.

Ethan! I can't let him see Rafe.

Turning my head, I search for Ethan and feel the badge being released. It thumps back against my blouse and swings like a pendulum.

When I swivel back to Rafe, he's gone. There's only empty space before me. It's like I saw a ghost who magically disappeared, evaporated into thin air. Rafe's absence is so sudden and disorienting that for a second I think I hallucinated the whole encounter, but then Ethan asks, "Who was that guy?"

61

"Tiffany?" Ethan's voice is questioning. "You okay?"

"What?" My mind is reeling from seeing Rafe.

"Who was that guy talking to you?" Ethan looks over my head to the spot where Rafe disappeared.

My mouth opens, but no words come out. How could I ever explain my childhood and those teenage years in Las Vegas? Ethan would never look at me the same way again. Would he regret kissing me if he knew? Would he walk away from me like Shelly and Rafe?

Not ready to risk it, I lie. "Oh, just some guy. He asked about the conference we're going to."

Easing the badge over my head, I take it off. "I forgot I was wearing this," I admit as I hold it out. The sun reflects glaringly off its plastic surface, sending rainbow beams of light spinning across our faces.

Ethan removes his conference badge. "I totally forgot, too." He folds the long lanyard into halves and then quarters before stuffing it in his pocket. "I can't believe we've been walking around like dorks all day wearing these." He laughs, the sound booming.

I wish I could share in his amusement, but a heavy sense of dread is growing in my stomach. I need to shake off the worry that seeing Rafe has generated in me.

Ethan plucks my badge out of my hand and rolls up the lanyard before placing it in his other pocket.

"What next? How about a drink?"

Still distracted, I nod.

We go to the teppanyaki restaurant in the Japan pavilion, where we order the signature drink, a Violet Sake. Ethan and I are in the bar area, full of families waiting for their tables.

It's loud, filled with the noise of people talking over one another and the shrieks of happy, overstimulated children. Kids dart in and out of their parents' legs, avoiding the reaching arms of adults who hope to calm them.

The Violet Sake is made from sake, lime, and purple pear juice. It has an electric purple color, similar to a grape Jolly Rancher. It tastes like a Jolly Rancher too, sweet and fruity. We sit close, knees and elbows touching, heads tilted together, so we can hear over the noise of the crowd and the background music of the bar.

I try to focus on what Ethan is saying, but it's difficult. My mind keeps replaying the moment when I saw Rafe. What's he doing here? How crazy that I bumped into him. It seems unlikely that we would be in the same place at the same time. No. This can't be a coincidence. Rafe's sudden appearance must have something to do with the weird text messages. But why didn't he say something? Where did he go? The questions go around and around with no answers to stop them.

Seeing Rafe brought back all those Las Vegas memories. Watching him walk away with Shelly had been one of the worst moments of my life, ranking only below the deaths of my mom and Mr. Chen. I've wondered for so long about what happened to Rafe and Shelly. Where they went and if they stayed together. When I picture them, it's no longer tinged with jealousy. It's more about hoping Shelly isn't alone, that she has someone to watch out for her.

It's stupid, but I wish I had asked Rafe about Shelly when I saw him today. If I could go back to that time and ask just one question, that would be it. *Is Shelly okay?* I'll probably never see Rafe again, though. Never find the answers to my past.

Ethan swirls the garish liquid in his glass with his straw, the lemon wedge and sprig of mint on top bumping into the edge of the cup with each rotation. He gives me an assessing look.

"So," he says slowly, "want to play a drinking game?"

Determined to stop thinking about Rafe, I welcome the distraction. "Sure. What did you have in mind? I doubt they'll let us play beer pong in here." I glance around at the crowded restaurant.

"No beer pong." Amber eyes move lightly over my face, studying me. "Let's play a game called Assumptions. I used to play it with my roommates back in college."

"Okay." I push away my memories. "How do you play?"

"It's easy. I make an assumption about you. If I'm right, you have to drink, but if I'm wrong, I take a drink. Then we switch, and you make an assumption about me."

I'm nervous about what secrets this game might uncover, but I agree. "I get it. Let's play."

"I'll start. You hated me the first time you met me." Ethan's gaze is steady, daring me to contradict him.

I grimace. "Hate is a strong word—"

He cuts me off. "It's either a yes or a no, a drink or not. No splitting hairs, Tiffy."

Reluctantly, I nod and take a long swallow of my sake but add, "I've changed my mind since then."

A lopsided smile plays across Ethan's face. "Good to hear," he says mildly. "Your turn."

I take a deep breath. "You hated me too the first time we met. I was rude to you."

His eyebrows lift in surprise. "First of all, it's not fair to repeat the same assumption, but I'll allow it since this misconception of yours needs to be cleared up. I most definitely didn't hate you the first time we met." He pauses and then firmly says, "Quite the opposite. Drink up because you were wrong."

Shocked into a momentary silence, I try to absorb what Ethan just told me. I really had believed he didn't like me. This new information makes me view all those initial interactions differently.

After a small sip, I tilt my glass at Ethan. "Your turn."

"You think I've had an easy life because of who my parents are and the sheltered, privileged suburbs where I was raised." His jaw is tight and defensive.

"No. I thought that when I very first met you, but I don't now. I understand how it can be a double-edged sword. How the decisions of your family that were made for you, decisions that you had no control over, can be a burden. It can force you into a mold that might not fit."

I think about Shelly and Brandi, about how scared Shelly was of someday turning into her mother. *Let me go, Tiffany.* I think about how Ethan wants to be different from his dad and brother, how he wants more than just a life working in the hospital.

What do *I* want that's different from what my mother had? The answer comes to me immediately, like it's been living in the back of my mind, waiting for this question.

I don't want to be alone.

I want a life filled with people and laughter, a husband, children, and friends. A full table on Thanksgiving, a home with crumpled wrapping paper and toys to assemble at Christmas. Summer vacations road-tripping in a car packed to the brim, heading to sandy beaches.

I want double dates with Melanie and midnight kisses with…Ethan? Is it too early to think about that? We've only shared one kiss, but when I picture that hazy future his face is the clearest thing I can see.

But how can Ethan be my future when he doesn't know about my past? This line of thought leads right back to Rafe, which is what I want to avoid the most.

"You drink, Ethan," I command.

"That's fair." His earlier tension is gone. My answer seemed to satisfy him. He takes a long draw from his sake drink. It's almost finished now.

"It's my turn." What should I ask next? It comes to me, something I've been wondering about. "You didn't think about me much during those five days that you didn't call after Cleveland." If I'm being honest, it still bothers me, those five long agonizing days.

A stormy expression moves over Ethan's face. "Wrong." His voice is harsher than I anticipated. "I thought about you *every* day. After being with you so much, it was like being in withdrawal."

His voice softens. "I missed you. Missed how you close your eyes when you take the first sip of coffee in the morning. Missed seeing the freckles on your nose after your makeup was washed off at night." Ethan leans back and folds his arms over his chest with a satisfied expression. "Since you know I thought about you, take a drink."

I swallow several sips in a row.

"I get to make the assumption now," Ethan reminds me. He taps his chin, thinking for a minute, and then smiles crookedly and says, "The kiss earlier today was the best you've ever had."

I pick up my glass and drain the rest of my drink, right down to the bottom. When I slam the empty glass on the bar, it rattles the drinks around us.

"Good," says Ethan as he polishes off his drink as well. "It was my best, too."

62

It's past 11:00 p.m., and the park has closed. On the bus ride back to the hotel, Ethan holds my hand, rubbing his thumb slowly over my knuckles as he looks out the window. There's a feeling of connection between us. It's an invisible string winding around, binding us together.

"Are you nervous about your big lecture tomorrow?" He leans his cheek against the top of my head.

"Yes," I answer honestly.

"You're going to be amazing," he says with quiet certainty. "You've been practicing for months."

All day the sky has promised a storm. As we pull up to the hotel, it finally delivers. Stuttering flashes of lightning are followed by low booms of thunder. A torrent of rain hits the ground so hard that raindrops bounce back up before falling to merge with the growing puddles on the concrete.

We run from the bus to the hotel. Ethan is right behind me, his hand on the small of my back, a bit of warmth on my otherwise cold body. Once inside the hotel, the air conditioning adds a chill to our rain-soaked skin, so Ethan and I quickly head up to my room.

He goes straight to the thermostat on the wall, cranking it up. There's a whoosh and that particular burnt plastic smell that comes from a heater when it's first turned on. A vent sits high in the ceiling. I move so I'm directly under it, hands up to catch the hot air spilling out like I'm warming myself at a campfire. Standing there soaking wet with my arms raised and back arched, I can feel my wet clothing cling to my body.

When I look at Ethan, I see him frozen in the doorway, staring at me with wide, hungry eyes full of heat as they roam over me, leaving a blazing trail that warms me from the inside out.

Breath catching in my throat, I watch as Ethan stalks across the room. His eyes are locked on me like he's a heat-seeking missile and I'm on fire. Once he reaches me, I place my hands on his chest. The warmth from his body sears through his wet clothing and leaks into my palms. Longing surges through me.

I want to be close to him. To know him, every inch inside and out. I long for him to know me, too. To stop hiding parts of myself. But I'm too scared and caught up in the moment to tell him about my past. I won't risk losing him, not tonight, when he's looking at me like this.

Like his heart is in my hands.

Ethan kisses me. This kiss isn't like the one on the pier. This one is fast and hard, overwhelming. As we continue to kiss, Ethan walks me slowly backward until I bump into the wall behind me. He pins me there, trapped like a butterfly under glass, between the wall and his hard chest, with no space between us. He places his hands on the wall on both sides of my head, leaning his full body weight against me.

Ethan bends his head to taste the hollow below my ear. He slides his mouth down my neck and kisses my collarbone. I move my head to the side to give him better access. Eventually, his mouth returns to mine.

When I kiss Ethan back, he gasps aloud. His chest is heaving. Then, he surprises me by pulling away, halting the kiss. Confused, I frown. I'm puzzled about why he made me stop something he was so obviously enjoying.

"Tiffy," he rasps out, "this isn't why I asked to come to Florida with you. I wasn't trying to trick you into kissing me."

"I know," I answer, stroking my hand down his arm.

Ethan sucks air through his teeth at my touch. "I don't want you to freak out tomorrow. If we kiss, you can't push me away," he warns, eyebrows lowered and face serious.

"I won't." I press against him. "I want this, Ethan. I've been thinking about it all day."

His laugh is almost humorless. "All day? I've been thinking about this since the moment we met." He grazes his nose along mine and whispers huskily, "You've got me shaken up like a bottle of champagne. Once you take that cork out, I won't be able to put it back in." Ethan pulls back and places his hand under my chin, tilting my head until I look him in the eye. His voice earnest, he says, "*Promise me*. Swear you won't run away."

"I promise," I whisper.

Those words are the release he's been waiting for. His hands are in my hair, his lips are on mine. It's intoxicating. We kiss some more, taking our time, moving slowly.

Ethan pulls away and searches my face. "You okay?" he whispers huskily.

All I can do is nod. Words are lost to me.

"Good girl," he whispers into the shell of my ear and kisses me again. It's dizzying how the blood rushes in my head and every nerve ending in my body responds like it's been lit up with dynamite.

Another kiss, this one harder. "Tiffy," Ethan breathes the name into my mouth with a wrenching gasp. I think about how I used to hate that nickname, but now it sounds like salvation, like a spell that can break the curse that hangs over me.

After a few more kisses, my eyelids grow heavy. Ethan notices right away and suggests we go to bed.

"Stay with me?" he asks, begging with his eyes. "Just sleep, I promise."

I agree and together we climb into the bed covered by a soft white comforter. Exhausted, wrung out by the excitement of the day, I don't just fall asleep. I tumble into it headfirst, but I'm not worried because I know Ethan will catch me.

There will be no nightmares tonight.

Only dreams coming true.

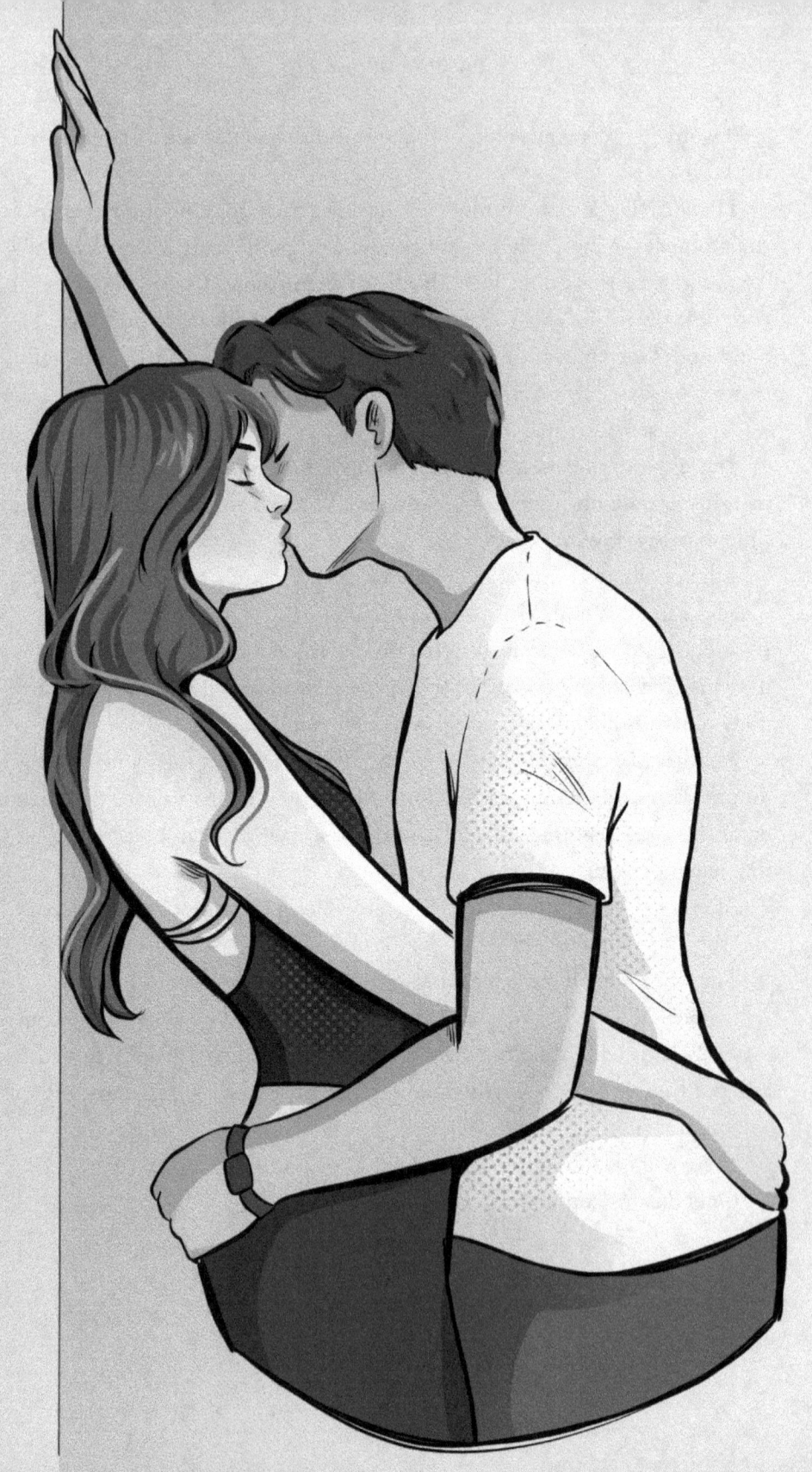

63

In the middle of the night, I wake and roll over to look at Ethan sleeping beside me. He's lying on his back, his boyish face peaceful. Long eyelashes cast shadows across his cheeks from the bright silver moonlight that cascades in through our hotel window. His arm is under my neck, a human pillow made just for me.

He took his shirt off before falling asleep. My eyes travel the length of him, from the well-defined muscles in his chest and arms to the hollow of his belly, the way his hip bones stick out all sharp and pointy. His skin glows as the light shifts over him, moving with his breath. I'm jealous of the moonlight, to kiss him everywhere at once as it does.

After our kissing earlier, I had fallen asleep so at peace, content in a way I've never felt before. Now, gazing at Ethan in that luminous silver light…it takes my breath away. There's a swelling in my chest like my heart is physically expanding to make room for him. I can't decide if it's a choice. Getting swept away by these feelings because now that I've touched him, the whole thing seems somehow inevitable. That it would be him for me and me for him.

When I trail kisses up his neck and end on his mouth, he rouses and sleepily looks at me. I continue to kiss him awake.

"What time is it?" Ethan asks, his voice raspy.

I peer at the red numbers lit up on the bedside clock. "A little past 3:00 a.m."

He sighs with pleasure. "This is a nice way to wake up."

I smile in the darkness. Then I bring my mouth to his in a soft kiss.

"You're insatiable, Tiffy."

"Insatiable?" I pull away, stung by his words. Does he think badly of me because I want to kiss him again? Am I being too forward? Too aggressive?

Ethan recognizes the hurt and insecurity in my voice. "No. No. Come back. That's not what I meant." His hand clamps around mine, and he pulls me until I'm lying on his chest.

He brushes the back of his hand lightly across my cheek. "I like it, waking up with you kissing me." A short, gentle laugh as his hand moves to my hair, tangling in it. "I mean a gorgeous woman in my bed waking me up for that. You're making teenage Ethan's dreams come true." He gives me a soft-sweet kiss.

"Really?" I'm still skittish.

"Really," he answers firmly, followed by another kiss, his tongue teasing mine.

Soothed, I ask, "What was teenage Ethan like?" I rest my chin on his chest, my hand rubbing lightly over his shoulder and down his arm.

Ethan shifts higher on the pillow so he can see me better. His eyes shine molten from the light through the window. "Teenage Ethan was afraid something like this would never happen." He chuckles. "I want to travel back in time, pat him on the head, and tell him don't worry, buddy, it's all going to work out. I was so worried back then about my parents and their expectations of me. Feeling like if I couldn't fit in with my family, then maybe I'd never fit in anywhere. Wondering if anyone could ever care for me just as I was." Squeezing my shoulder lightly, he grins at me. "Wondering if I'd ever get to touch a girl."

He drags me farther up his body until we're eye to eye. He kisses me again. This time it's a spine-tingling, toe-curling type of kiss.

He continues, his voice low and rough, "I want to tell teenage Ethan that he's going to meet this incredible woman whose brains and beauty and strength are going to blow his mind."

My mouth is on his, and we kiss endlessly.

Eventually, we grow tired. I roll away from him. Ethan spoons me and runs his fingers over and over through my long hair as he whispers into my ear, "You're mine now. *All mine.*" There's something primal in his voice, something fierce, possessive, and unyielding. Those are the last words I hear before I slip into a fathomless ocean of sleep.

64

The next morning, I wake and lie still with my eyes closed, replaying the events from last night. I linger on the way Ethan kissed me and the sweet things he said. Without opening my eyes, I reach out and run my hand across the bed to where he should be.

When my hand encounters nothing, just a pillow empty and cold, my heart gives a frightened spasm. Eyes open, I search for him, my fingers sweeping over the sheets even though I can clearly see that his side of the bed is empty.

That's when I find the note on my nightstand, propped up against the table lamp.

Tiffy,

Off to the gym.

Be back to pick you up at 8 a.m.

Ethan

PS Last night was the best night.

The postscript line makes me smile, a grin that feels almost too big for my face. I'm so happy that I might shatter and, if I did, pure joyful sunlight would surely come streaming out of all my broken cracks. That's how Ethan makes me feel.

While I'm brushing my teeth, worry chips away at that happiness. My brain begins its usual laundry list of questions. I wonder if it'll be awkward with Ethan when he comes back from the gym. What will happen when we go back to Columbus? The scariest question of all—how to tell him about my past?

Even though I'm terrified that telling Ethan about my history in Las Vegas will change how he looks at me, he deserves the truth. If I really want this relationship to have a chance, which I *really, really* do, I need to come clean. I resolve to talk with him after the conference today.

My phone dings with an incoming text.

Melanie: Good luck with UR presentation.

Tiffany: Thanks.

Melanie: What time R U giving it?

Tiffany: Nine-thirty. Hoping if I do a good job, it'll get back to Dr. Washburn. Maybe I'll finally get that Resident of the Month award.

Melanie: U better, or I'm going on strike!

Tiffany: Lol. Appreciate the support.

Melanie: Always.

"Tiffy, I'm here," Ethan calls out as the hotel room door slams closed behind him. I'd given him my extra room key earlier.

"In the bathroom," I call back as I frown in the mirror, fumbling with the clasp of my necklace.

"Hey you." He enters the room and smiles when he meets my eyes in the mirror. He reaches around me to place a large iced latte on the bathroom counter. I don't have to taste it to know it's vanilla.

"Thanks." Smiling, I lift my gaze and take in his face, clean-shaven and so very handsome. My eyes drop to his lips. My cheeks burn as I remember all the kisses we shared last night.

Noticing that I'm struggling with the necklace, Ethan comes up close behind. "Here, let me help with that." Gently, he takes the metal chain out of my hands. As I hold my hair out of the way, he bends close and fastens the necklace, letting it fall to rest between my breasts.

"Good morning." His breath is warm on the nape of my neck as he presses a kiss to my sensitive skin. That touch sends tingles of longing traveling along the highway of nerves throughout my body.

I turn until I'm facing him. "Morning."

Ethan doesn't move away, so we're pressed close together, the small of my back braced against the sink behind me. Lifting my chin, I kiss him deeply. It feels so good to touch him. I could live in this moment, stay here forever. With Herculean effort, I drag my mouth away from his.

"We need to get down to the conference. It'll start soon."

Ethan presses harder against me. "What conference?" he jokes.

My hand is firm against his shoulder as I laughingly push him away. "Come on now. You know what conference. The one downstairs about to start in, oh," I check my watch, "ten minutes."

"We could skip the first lectures. Just go down when it's time for you to give your talk," Ethan says hopefully, resisting my attempts to move him out of my way.

"We skipped out yesterday. We can't keep missing the lectures," I insist, shaking my finger at him. "There's a nuclear medicine cardiac imaging presentation at 9:00 that I want to see."

With a dramatic sigh, he lowers his forehead until it rests against mine. "Who would have thought I'd fall for such a rule follower?" He shoves himself away and turns and walks out of the bathroom.

"I got a little something for you," he calls back over his shoulder.

"You did?" I follow him into the bedroom, practically bouncing up and down in my excitement to see what he's brought.

His body blocks my view as he picks something up off the desk. He hides it behind his back and grins at me mischievously.

"What is it?" I peek around his tall frame, trying unsuccessfully to see what he's holding.

With a loud "Surprise!" Ethan produces a gorgeous bouquet of long-stem red roses surrounded by babies' breath. The flowers' lush aroma fills the room.

"Ethan!" I exclaim as he hands me the blossoms. "They're beautiful." I press my nose to the scarlet petals and inhale deeply. "They smell like heaven. You didn't have to do that."

"I know I didn't have to, but I wanted to." He smiles crookedly. "They have a gift shop downstairs, and as soon as I saw them I thought of you. The red reminded me of your hair." He reaches out and runs a strand through his fingers. "Plus, I wanted to give you something to say good luck on your presentation. You're going to rock it."

With the flowers in one hand, I wrap my other arm around him in a hug. "Thank you," I murmur into his chest.

He's so tall that it's easy for him to place a kiss on the crown of my head and then rest his cheek there. "What have you done to me, Tiffy? I want to buy you flowers and chocolates in a heart-shaped box." His rueful laugh rumbles through my skull. "I hardly recognize myself, but I like it."

I fill the hotel ice bucket with water and carefully place the flowers in it, arranging the stems so they spread out evenly.

After a few more lingering kisses, Ethan and I gather our things to head downstairs to the conference.

As 9:30 a.m. grows closer, my nerves ratchet up higher and higher. *T3b, T3b, T3b,* I mentally chant, determined to get it right this time. Before I know it, it's time for my lecture. I ascend the steps and approach the podium. With microphone in hand, I begin my presentation. The slides click by as I go through the renal cancer case.

"Given that this patient's cancer ascended into the inferior vena cava but remained below the level of the diaphragm," I say, "his cancer stage is T3b."

Yes! Nailed it.

With that out of the way, the rest of my presentation will be smooth sailing.

Ethan's triumphant smile slices through the rest of the anonymous faces in the crowd. He does a mini fist-pump motion with his hand, which makes me grin. Even though I hadn't told him I was worried about messing up that part of my lecture, he had known. That's how well he understands me. It's a special thing, to be seen and accepted like that.

Focusing on my presentation, I continue. "I'm happy to report that this patient recently had his follow-up CAT scan and remains cancer-free. We will continue to monitor—"

The door at the back of the lecture hall bangs opens, letting in a shaft of light that shines directly into my eyes, blinding me. I pause, momentarily disoriented. It takes a second to blink away the bright spots that remain as the door closes. Once my vision clears, I see the figure of a man who just walked into my conference.

A green-eyed man who obviously doesn't belong.

Rafe.

65

Time slows down as I stare through the crowd to the back of the room. I have two thoughts in rapid succession.

Thought one is: *What is Rafe doing here?*

Followed by thought two: *Ethan!*

Ethan and Rafe together in the same room are enough to give me a heart attack. I search through the dark until I find Ethan in the audience. He's looking up at me with a concerned frown, no doubt wondering why my lecture came to an abrupt standstill. He hasn't noticed Rafe yet. I'm worried that if Ethan sees Rafe, he'll recognize him from Epcot yesterday. I need to get Rafe out of here before that happens.

But first, my lecture. I clear my throat and stutter. "Excuse me…um…as I was saying, we will continue to…um, monitor."

I glance up, distracted by Rafe's grim presence. The scowl on his face speaks volumes. My mouth goes dry as panic hijacks my brain. I stare into the crowd and a sea of unfamiliar faces looks back as I fumble with my computer, trying to advance to the next slide. Too many eyes on me, their weight heavy. Too many of my colleagues are watching me fail.

"Monitor this patient every six months for reoccurrence…" I swallow so loudly that the microphone picks up the sound. Another flick of my eyes shows Rafe hasn't budged. His arms are crossed over his chest. His wide-legged stance suggests he's an immovable object.

Warning sirens of alarm blare in the back of my head. I cough into my fist. "That…um, concludes my presentation. I'd be happy to answer any questions."

A couple of hands shoot into the air, and I mentally curse them. Keeping my false smile in place and deliberately not looking at either Rafe or Ethan, I answer their questions with brief responses.

Once that's done, I say a hasty "thank you" and take my leave as the audience applauds. I barely hear them clapping, too overwhelmed by anxiety.

Heart in my throat, I rush down the aisle, heading to Ethan. As I approach, he stands with a huge smile and congratulations on his lips. Before he can speak, I mouth "bathroom" to him and veer off toward the back doors of the conference room.

It breaks my heart to see that beautiful smile fall from his face and to watch his arms drop by his side, but I don't want to draw attention to him. I'm hoping Rafe doesn't know who Ethan is and doesn't know he's here.

Once I've walked past Ethan, I look over to Rafe. His expression is openly hostile, causing my stomach to lurch heavily. We make eye contact, and he flicks his eyes at the exit, telling me to follow.

When I push open the doors, Rafe is waiting in the lobby.

"How did you find me?" My voice is suddenly hoarse.

To answer, Rafe grabs the badge from my chest and holds it up for me to see. There it is. My name and the name of the conference. I hadn't thought about how easy it would be for him to track me down with that information.

Holding my badge, Rafe says, "I called your hospital in Columbus. They said you are here in Orlando for a conference. I didn't know which one. I was figuring it out when I bumped into you yesterday. This told me the rest."

"I don't understand." I'm confused, attempting to grasp how he ended up here. "What were you doing at Epcot? Did you decide to take a day off from stalking me to go to an amusement park?"

"I have an old contact, one who's good at hacking into hotel reservation systems. He works at Epcot. I was going to have him figure out where you are staying, but then I saw you and this." He tugs the lanyard lightly. His laugh is low and gravelly, fingers racked across wet sand. "Isn't that quite the coincidence, Tiffany? For me to find you there? It's like fate wants us reunited. To finish what we started."

I yank the badge out of his hands and look around surreptitiously. Between gritted teeth, I hiss, "What are you talking about?"

Fury grips me. This was supposed to be *my* moment of victory. I successfully finished my presentation. Ethan and I are together. I was happy for once. Finally letting go of my fear, my pain, my past. But here comes Rafe, set to destroy all I've built. Ready to drag me down yet again.

A quick glance around the room shows that only one hotel worker is here, busy cleaning up the remainder of the breakfast buffet. He doesn't appear to be listening to our conversation, but, just to be safe, I point away from the lobby where we stand. "Let's talk over there."

"Fine." Rafe languidly picks up a black backpack that's been sitting by his feet and throws it over his shoulder. He's moving too slow for my taste, so I grab him by the upper arm and drag him away. It feels weird to touch him. His arm is so big and muscular that it's foreign to me. I still think of him as the teenage boy I used to know. This new version of Rafe is disorienting and scary.

Earlier, I had noticed an alcove off the conference lobby, the kind where you go for privacy to make a phone call. This is where I take him. The space is small, forcing us to stand close together. It has two old-fashioned–looking telephones mounted on the back wall, with their cords dangling down.

Once we step in, I whirl around to confront him. "What do you want?" I snap, speaking quietly so people passing by can't hear. There's no door here. We can still be seen, but at least we're out of the line of sight for people entering and exiting the lecture hall.

He doesn't bother with the niceties. "Money or, more specifically, diamonds."

"What?! Are you crazy? I don't have any diamonds." It's a struggle to keep my voice down. I'm so outraged. "I'm a resident. I make less than minimum wage." Rafe is barking up the wrong tree if he thinks he'll get rich off me. I've got more student debt than anything else. After I pay for this trip, I'll have less than $100 dollars left in my bank account.

He gives me a look like I'm stupid. "Not from you. From Shelly."

"What do you mean from Shelly?" I glance around, out of my depth. "Is she here?" I wouldn't be surprised to see Shelly waltz into the room at this point. If one ghost is back to haunt me, why not two?

Rafe runs a hand through his thick dark hair, looking frustrated. "Shelly's not here, but she had diamonds, ones that we took from Johnny's place. She hid them, wanted to keep them for herself."

"Hid them? Where?"

"At the Starlight."

The Starlight. A place I've visited in my nightmares so very often.

Little bird, where are you?

"I thought they destroyed that place. Weren't there plans to implode it?" I picture the decrepit building in my mind. It was run-down back when I was in high school, so it must be a total disaster by now. How's it even standing?

"The politicians have been battling over it for years, so the Starlight's still there, just waiting for us." There's a greedy glint in his eyes.

I stare at him with bewilderment, trying to wrap my mind around his plan. "How do you know Shelly was telling the truth? If you guys were fighting, she could've been messing with you."

Rafe shakes his head vehemently and says, "No. I saw those diamonds in the duffle bag with my own eyes when we first got to the Starlight before you showed up."

"Why didn't you go back for them right then?" I spit out.

"I didn't notice that they were missing until later. By then, we were so far away it didn't make sense to go back. But now it does."

"Why?" I question.

He sets his jaw. "I owe some guys."

"What does that have to do with me?" I glare at him, angry at how adversarial this conversation has been. So much for "Nice to see you. How have you been?"

"Shelly told me I'd never find the diamonds." Rafe takes a step closer. "But she didn't know that I have a secret weapon."

"What's your secret weapon?" I fling my hands up in the air.

"*You* are, Tiffany. You're my secret weapon."

I scoff. "How? I don't know where Shelly put them. I didn't even know they existed until a minute ago."

"You know Shelly better than anyone, better than her own mother." He's moved during our conversation, subtly angling himself until he's in front of the doorway. Blocking my only way of escape with his large body.

There's something menacing about the new Rafe. A hardness to him that goes beyond the massive amount of muscle he's acquired since I last saw him. "You're going to go with me and find those diamonds. *Right now.* We're running out of time."

"No way." My voice becomes louder, almost yelling. I can't believe this man's audacity. "Why on earth would I help you?"

Rafe puts his hand in his pocket. For a terrifying minute I think he's going to pull out a gun, but instead he takes out a small square object. "Because if you don't come with me now," he says in a deadly serious voice, "I'm going to walk into that fancy conference room. I'm going to rip the microphone out of the speaker's hands and tell them all about how you used to work the Strip and how you lied and stole. Then I'm going to put this on the projector so the entire room can see exactly who you really are." He holds up the object for me to see, just out of my reach.

It's a Polaroid photo, worn dim and dirty with age, of two young girls grinning widely with their arms slung around each other, one in a revealing white angel costume and the other dressed as a sexy red devil.

Me and Shelly.

The photo we took the first night we worked the Strip together. Shelly must have kept it, and somehow Rafe got his hands on it. Heart sinking, I stare at the Polaroid. It's clearly me, and it's damning. If it's shown at the conference, I can kiss my career good-bye. Bad enough that Ethan would see it, but I could at least talk to him, try to explain. He's a kind man who might understand and forgive me.

It's the several hundred other doctors in that room who are the problem. Doctors who in a few years I'll need to hire me and to work beside me. If this picture gets out, my reputation will be permanently damaged. No one will want to work with me. I'll always be known as that show-girl doctor who did terrible things, criminal things, in Las Vegas.

"We're leaving right now," says Rafe. "There's a plane to Vegas in one hour. You're going to buy tickets for both of us. If we hurry, we can make it."

"I don't have enough money." I back away, with my hands raised, only to run into the wall behind me.

I'm trapped.

"That's what credit cards are for," he argues. "And don't tell me that you don't have one because I saw you use it in Epcot."

His words chill me. How long had Rafe been watching me yesterday?

"I can't do it," I argue, not yet ready to give in to this crazy scheme. "I have to get back to the conference. People in there are expecting me. They'll notice if I'm gone too long."

He huffs, "Who'll notice? Your boyfriend?"

"He's not my boyfriend." A powerful urge to protect Ethan at all costs overcomes me. I can't let Rafe drag him into this madness. My past mistakes can't be Ethan's downfall.

Rafe quirks one eyebrow at me. "Oh yeah? You kiss all your friends like that?"

Shoot.

That answers that question. Rafe had been watching long enough yesterday to see me kiss Ethan on the pier. He knows who Ethan is and what he means to me. I can't let him leverage that knowledge to hurt Ethan. I just can't.

Rafe takes one step closer to me and then two. "I remember once upon a time when you kissed me like that, Tiffany." His voice is soft, but his eyes are hard. "Maybe your boyfriend would like to hear about that kiss as well."

"Shut up," I snap, which sparks grim satisfaction in his eyes.

"You know what? Now that I think about it, not only will I mention your name when I get up on that stage, I'll call out your boyfriend, too." Rafe puts the final nail in my coffin. "What's his name? Ethan? Dr. Ethan Clark." A cruel smile at my look of disbelief. "You weren't the only one wearing a name tag yesterday."

My stomach sinks into the ground.

"We leave now." Rafe adjusts the backpack straps on his shoulders.

"No." I cross my arms over my chest, belligerent.

"Yes. Or else I walk through those doors and spill all your secrets. Oh, and don't bother trying to call the police or anyone else for help because a good friend of mine is holding a copy of this photo and has instructions to post it all over the web if something happens to me." He takes a threatening step closer. "I'm not letting this go. Not until I get my way."

I stand there, indecisive, fear thickening in my throat.

"Come on, Tiffany," he urges. "A smart woman like you should know you can't outrun your past. Trust me, I've tried."

I look longingly across the room, at the large wooden doors that lead back into the safety of the conference. The current guest speaker's voice echoes faintly through the closed doors, but it might as well be in another universe.

It's agony, having Ethan a room away. I want so badly to go to him. To tell him about Rafe and what I'm being asked to do. For so long, I've been on my own. Able to handle my problems with no one else to help. Now, after one night with Ethan, I want nothing more than to burst through the doors and run into his arms. How nice it would be to offer all these problems to him and then solve them together.

But I don't go to Ethan. My mom taught me that sometimes love is about sacrifice. Giving away parts of yourself to keep the person you care about happy and safe. At that moment, it hits me with crystal clarity.

I love Ethan.

Maybe it's too early to feel this way about him, or maybe my brain is just catching up to what my heart already knows. Either way, it's the truth. I love him and will do anything for him.

I book the plane tickets on my phone and leave with Rafe.

66

PRESENT, LAS VEGAS, NEVADA

Desolate, I stare out of the airplane window, watching the clouds wisp by as the plane levels off from takeoff. All I can think about is Ethan. I can't believe it took me this long to see the truth.

I love him.

In my romance books, sometimes love is a bludgeon that hits you over the head. But now I see love can also be like a thief in the night, sneaking in through a crack in the window and slipping into your bed. That's what my love for Ethan is like. It snuck up on me.

But can he ever love me, the *real* me, back? If he finds out all the awful things I've done…

It won't matter, anyway. When I don't return from the bathroom, Ethan will think I broke my promise. The one thing he asked of me was not to run away, but that is *exactly* what this will look like. He'll never forgive me.

I need to stop thinking about Ethan and focus on my safety. I don't understand Rafe's plans yet. What will he do to me if I find the diamonds? What will he do if I fail? Determined to find some answers, I break the tense silence that has existed between Rafe and me since we left the hotel.

First, the question I wanted to ask yesterday. "Where is Shelly? Is she okay?"

Rafe is so big and muscular that his upper body extends into my space. When his elbow touches my arm, he jerks away. "Last time I saw Shelly, she was in Mexico and she was fine. You always worried too much about her."

A new thought occurs to me. "How do you know she hasn't already come back and claimed the diamonds? Maybe she beat you there?"

"She wouldn't go to Vegas." Rafe gives a humorless laugh. "Shelly's got a warrant out for her arrest. She can't risk coming back into the United States."

"A warrant? For what?" I sit up straight, alarmed.

"Don't worry about it," is all he'll say. Rafe's not in a very conversational mood, but then he's always been that way.

I'm not going to let him off the hook so easily. Some things have bothered me for years, and now that I've got him trapped in a seat next to me for a couple of hours I'll force him to speak, somehow.

I take my time and observe him. He's tense, all tight jaw and frowning mouth. There are lines on his face that he didn't used to have, little wrinkles in the corners of his eyes and bracketing his mouth. Not laugh lines, more like worry lines. I'm guessing life hasn't been easy since he left Las Vegas.

"Did you plan it all along? Taking the money and abandoning me? Whose idea was it? Yours or Shelly's?" Bitterness fills my words. It curls poisonous around each syllable. I've waited for so long to ask that question.

Surprisingly, he answers. "It was all Shelly. She was the mastermind, planned the whole thing." He gives me a shrewd glance. "You always underestimated her. Besides, we gave you some money. We didn't take it all."

"A small fraction of the money and then you left." I shake my head. "Anyway, we shouldn't have done it. We shouldn't have taken it."

"Yeah, but we did, and I bet you used that money, even though it was dirty." A knowing look from him. "Didn't you?"

My silence is all the admission Rafe needs. A cruel, satisfied smile expands across his face. "Thought so."

I almost argue with him, explaining how I had no choice. How after my mother died, that money was the only way to get free of her medical debt. But I stay quiet because it's a lie.

There's always a choice.

"It was still wrong," I persist. "I shouldn't have done it. I especially regret lying to Stewart. He deserved better than that." There's the bitter sting of tears in the back of my throat, but I won't let Rafe see me cry.

"You lied to Stewart, and we lied to you. On and on, that's how it goes. Welcome to the real world, Tiffany. It's not all rainbows and sunshine. Everybody lies." He's matter of fact about it, like this is some universal truth he's explaining.

I don't buy it. Ethan's never lied to me. He's proven that not everyone takes from each other without giving back. My mother and Mr. Chen weren't like that either. Rafe may live in a pessimistic world, but it doesn't have to be my reality. For years, I've lived isolated from other people, scared of exactly that. I refuse to live that way any longer.

He continues, "I used to feel bad for you. I knew what you were going through with your mom, but now I don't feel sorry for you anymore. Look at you. Living this sweet life you've made for yourself." Jealousy colors Rafe's cheeks a blotchy red. "While I've been on the run this whole time. We were both there that night. We both did the crime, but I'm the one who paid. The way I figure, you owe me."

His eyes glitter with malice. The boy I once knew is gone, replaced by a resentful and angry man. "That's why I started sending you those text messages."

I gasp. "That was you?" I figured it was him or Shelly, but still the admission rocks me. All these past months I've been tortured, wondering, worrying about those messages. Who sent them and what they meant.

It was *him*. Rafe. He was behind it all along.

He nods. "I could tell you'd deliberately forgotten us. Buried your past. I need you to get a shovel and dig it back up. I wanted to trigger your memories. You're going to find those diamonds for me. I'll retire to some tiny island and drink pina coladas for the rest of my life." He has a distant expression, like he's picturing this idyllic future.

"And if I can't find the diamonds?" I counter.

Rafe moves faster than a cobra striking, his face suddenly in front of mine. "There's no *if*. You better find them." I shrink back against my seat, retreating from the fury I see in his eyes. "You'll be punished if you fail. If you don't believe me, well, you obviously didn't know who I was back then and you sure don't understand who I've become now."

For the first time, I'm truly afraid of him.

67

When I pull the rental car into the Starlight parking lot, the sense of déjà vu is so vivid that I expect to look over and see Shelly in her devil costume sitting next to me. But there's no Shelly, only a glowering Rafe.

There are fewer cars in the lot now, and some of them appear abandoned, like they've been here for years. These cars lean drunkenly, their black tires slouching deflated against the ground. Weeds grow out of cracks in the asphalt and, grasping, clamber their way up into the cars' rotted undercarriages.

Rusted and dented No Trespassing signs cling to bent wire fencing.

The building also looks more worn. Only a few windows on the uppermost floors remain intact. The rest are shattered, with jagged glass lining their edges like the gnashing teeth of some terrible monster.

I could swear the whole structure leans drunkenly to the left. A wing of hotel rooms on the west end has completely collapsed. That side of the building is flayed open, its outer walls crumbled away, so the floors have fallen on top of each other like layers in a rotten cake. A barricade is in front of the building, a concrete half wall, easy to climb over, with a red and black sign that says "Danger, Keep Out."

"Are you sure it's safe to go inside?" I fidget nervously, staring between the sign and the fractured casino. "It doesn't seem structurally sound."

A grunt is all I get in response. Rafe's head is down as he digs through his backpack. Like a messed-up version of Mary Poppins, he pulls out two long heavy-duty flashlights and hands one to me. I resist the urge to hit him on the back of the head with it. Pretty sure I could knock him unconscious. How good that would feel, to have the reverberations from the blow travel up my arm. To watch him slump to the ground and then run for help, screaming.

But I don't.

Who knows if this mysterious person who holds a second copy of my show-girl picture even exists? But if they do and they post the photo like Rafe threatens, I'll end up in a worse position.

No. Better to give him what he wants and then plead to be released.

Rafe didn't used to be a killer…at least not as far as I knew.

As soon as we enter the Starlight, I realize where Shelly hid the diamonds.

Little bird.

It's so obvious that I almost doubt myself. Surely Shelly wouldn't have hidden them some place I know so well? But how would she have ever guessed that Rafe would contact me? Find me and bring me with him to search for the treasure. When Shelly last saw Rafe and me together, their betrayal had devastated me. She probably assumed I'd never willingly help him. Which is true—there is nothing willing about this. Rafe keeps one hand on my arm as we enter the Starlight as if he doesn't trust me not to run away.

The hotel is in shambles. Heaps of rubble and debris line the hallways. Off-kilter doors have broken free of their hinges, hanging at awkward angles. The old, patterned carpet is wet from rain that has blown in through broken windows. It squelches under foot. The whole place smells like rot and decay. I stifle a cough in my throat, putting the back of my hand over my nose to block the stench.

Rafe doesn't seem to be bothered by any of it. He eagerly scans the rooms as we walk past, searching for a clue about the diamonds' location. The flashlight's beam skitters over the walls and floor as he swings it from side to side. Still clutching my arm, he drags me ever deeper into the hotel.

There's a new-looking rectangular box in one hallway. It has a diamond-shaped orange sign on the side showing a picture of a ball with a jagged crack through its middle and lines radiating out from its sides. Like a bomb exploding. Rafe walks right past it, but it catches my eye. I halt to take a closer look, holding my ground even as he tugs on my arm, urging me forward.

"Hey." I yank back, countering his pull. "What's this?"

"Beats me. Let's get going," Rafe says gruffly, not bothering to glance at the box. He jerks harder on me, but I dig my heels into the soft carpet, rooting myself into the floor.

"No. Tell me what this is. What am I looking at?" I should already know the answer, but my mind doesn't want to comprehend what my eyes are seeing.

"It's probably dynamite or C3," Rafe admits as he stops tugging on me.

"Why would they have that kind of explosive in here?" My heart hammers in my chest, trying madly to escape my rib cage.

"Because they're going to blow this place up." He almost looks guilty. "The City Council finally reached an agreement with the owners. They want to clear this land to make way for a new luxury resort."

"What?" My voice rises, pitching into a panicked tone. "When?"

"Tonight," he answers reluctantly. "They plan to broadcast it on TV. It will be a big show."

"What?! Are you kidding me?" I'm shouting now. "Why aren't there police cars out front to stop stupid people like us from coming in?"

"I dunno." He shrugs. "I expected we'd have a lot more trouble getting in here. They've been talking about the demolition for weeks, so maybe they thought that was enough of a deterrent for most people. This is why we had to come today. Don't you see, Tiffany? It's my last chance to get those diamonds."

Suddenly motivated to find the gems and escape, I spin around, trying to get my bearings. It had been hectic when Shelly and I were chased into the hotel by those awful, scary men. My mind was so overcome with fear back then that I worry I won't be able to find the small storage room again.

I turn in a circle. A hallway looks familiar. I start toward it, but stop. "How do I know you'll let me go if I help?" I ask quietly.

"If we find the diamonds, then that's it. That'll be the last time you ever see me," Rafe promises, his gaze steady.

"But how do I *know*?" I insist.

I want to believe him.

When we were young, I'd trusted Rafe, maybe because he had rescued me or maybe because I felt like he kept a protective eye on Shelly and me. Even though I knew he did bad things, illegal things, there was something in him that I had found comforting.

After he and Shelly left, I thought I had been delusional, attributing Rafe with a noble heart he didn't deserve. Now I find myself asking those same questions.

Who is Rafe? Savior? Protector? Betrayer? Friend or Foe?

"Because I said so." He sets his jaw.

I stare into his eyes, looking for the truth. It's like gazing into a murky pond. Things slip and slither beneath the surface, but I can't make out their form. As usual, I can't decipher his intentions.

"You'll just have to believe me, Tiffany." He pinches the bridge of his nose. "I understand why you don't trust me, but there's nothing I can do about that. We're running out of time. If you want to get back to your doctor life, see that boyfriend of yours, there's only one choice for you to make. Let's go." He doesn't move toward me, doesn't grab me or force me.

Rafe waits for me to decide.

"Fine," I say, still angry and unsure but unable to think of a better solution. Pointing to the hallway that looks promising, I tell him, "I'm not positive, but it might be down there."

Rafe lets out a breath, and his shoulders slump. In the irregular beam from our flashlights, he appears older than his age. His posture is stooped, and his arms hang heavy at his sides. As I walk away, I almost miss his whispered, "Thank you."

We wander through the hotel, turning this way and that, an uneasy truce between us. Rafe helps me, holding me steady as we clamber over a pile of old bed frames that someone has shoved together to make a wall-like barrier in one corridor.

I wrack my memories as we move along, trying to recall that terrifying sprint with Shelly. It's been so long, but the experience was traumatizing enough to form an indelible mark on my mind. The route to the supply room comes back to me in bits and pieces.

Finally, I reach what I think is the right door, but the door frame is warped. The door is jammed shut. Rafe puts his shoulder against it and, muscles straining, gives a mighty shove. The door flies open, and we enter. It's dark as night in the room. I use my flashlight to search around.

There it is.

In the ceiling is the faint outline of the square-shaped hatch. Just like I remembered. The room has been cleaned out since I last saw it. The cardboard boxes and supplies were taken away. It's an empty shell now, completely bare inside.

"Up there," I tell Rafe, pointing to the hatch with my light. "I think that's where Shelly might have hidden the diamonds."

He bends back, hands on his hips, and squints up at it. "How do we reach it?"

"Don't know. When I was here before, we stood on some boxes, but they're gone now." I tap my foot, impatient. How long will it take to figure this out? How long until those explosives go off? The longer I stand here, the greater the sense of urgency I feel. A clock is ticking down in my head.

"I think I saw a chair out in the hallway. Hang on." Rafe disappears for a minute and returns holding a plastic folding chair. He positions it directly under the opening and stands on it. Lifting his arms above his head, he stretches toward the hatch but can't reach it. Growling in frustration, he gets down and drops his hands back to his side.

He gives me a pleading look, asking for help.

"Lift me up," I command as I place my flashlight on the ground, angling it to light up the small room.

Rafe's eyebrows knit together in confusion. "What?" The lines in his face are exaggerated from my flashlight. His shadow looms huge on the wall behind him, looking like an ogre brought to life.

Quickly, I move in front and stand with my back to him. I lift my arms up over my head. "Pick me up. Hopefully, I can reach the opening if you lift me high enough."

Rafe places his hands under my arms. With a grunt, he lifts me high in front of him. It's not enough.

"Put me on your shoulders."

Raising me even higher, he sets me on his shoulders. He climbs back up on the chair. I wobble, avoiding falling only by grabbing onto his head. He hisses as I yank, pulling out strands of hair.

After a minute, we steady. I balance, sitting on his shoulders, and stretch my arms out as far as I can. My fingertips graze the hatch and then I get purchase. I can fully touch it now. Bracing one hand on the ceiling, I push up against the wood door. It lifts easily, swinging away and falling into the attic space with a loud thump.

"A little higher." Straining, I grasp the splintered wooden frame of the opening. He rises on his toes, and I pull myself up, using every upper body muscle I have. Rafe curses as my flailing foot kicks him in the head. Wiggling my legs, I slowly army crawl forward until I'm fully inside.

Rafe shouts from below, "Do you see it?" His hand is clasped on his forehead, rubbing the spot where my shoe connected with his skull.

I retrieve my phone from my pocket, relieved it didn't fall out in my struggle. When I was here before with Shelly, we had been too scared to use our lights, so I'm not sure what to expect.

Shining the light around, I see that it's a cramped space with low ceilings. Box-like metal air conditioning ductwork and snaking bundles of electrical wires take up the bulk of the area. A thick layer of dust lies over everything. The beam of my light illuminates delicate cobwebs, turning them silver and throwing their lacy shadows along the walls.

Far from the opening, tucked behind a stud, is a dirty plastic bag with a faded red K-Mart logo on the side. It's out of place in the otherwise utilitarian space. Crouching, I carefully make my way over to it, trying to put my weight only on the wooden support beams and not on the thin layers of drywall between them. The last thing I need right now is to fall through the ceiling and break a leg. Not while that imaginary explosive timer ticks down in my head.

Balanced carefully on one of the beams, I hold my phone with one hand and use the other to open the plastic bag. The light reflects off the faceted glittering stones inside. I gasp at the sight.

It's diamonds.

Lots and lots of diamonds.

68

The diamonds sparkle and glimmer. They're so beautiful that I want to push my hands into them. I want to bathe in them, to swim in them. Instead, I seal the bag, tying a knot on top.

When I faintly hear my name called, I assume it's Rafe yelling from below. Seconds later, I realize that's not Rafe's voice. That sounds like…Ethan?

"Tiffany," Ethan shouts, closer now, panic pushing his voice an octave higher.

"Ethan! Ethan! I'm here." I scramble across the support beams, but I'm still far away from the opening when incoherent arguing erupts from the room beneath me. Muffled thumps and crashing noises follow. When I finally reach the edge of the hatch door, I'm shocked by the view below.

Ethan and Rafe face off, circling each other like angry wolves. Judging by their panting breaths and the trickle of blood seeping from Ethan's brow into his eye, this fight has been going on for a while.

As I watch in horror, Rafe lunges at Ethan, his meaty forearms grabbing only air as Ethan drops to the ground and sweeps his leg out to trip Rafe. It works. Arms flailing, Rafe falls backward, but he bounces up quickly.

Rafe charges at Ethan with his head down like a battering ram. Ethan neatly sidesteps him and catches his arm as he runs past. Using Rafe's arm for leverage, Ethan swings him back toward him and puts out his elbow, which collides with Rafe's belly.

Rafe doubles over his wounded stomach, gasping for air. Clutching his abdomen and glaring at Ethan, Rafe dances sideways, light on the balls of his feet, moving like a professional boxer.

Ethan holds his ground, his knees and arms bent in the classic karate ready pose. I recognize it from his morning workouts.

"Ethan! Rafe! Stop!" I shout.

Rafe and Ethan don't respond to my plea. The men are too busy battling to hear me, or they're deliberately ignoring me. Either way, I need them to quit fighting before someone gets seriously hurt.

The only way to get down from the attic space is to drop from the ceiling, but it's a long fall. I'm worried I'll break a bone. Indecisive, I gnaw on my lip as the fight below continues.

Rafe is the more aggressive fighter of the two men. He closes the distance and ducks under Ethan's arm to punch him in the ribs.

The wind whooshes out of Ethan as he stumbles from the heavy blow. Rafe follows Ethan's retreat, sending out a volley of fist punches, one of which lands on Ethan's back and another on the side of his head.

Ethan sways unsteadily as he circles to the left. Blood streams in a steady rivulet from his brow into his eye. He brushes the blood away with the back of his hand and flicks it to the floor.

Chest heaving, Rafe brings his fists up higher, preparing for another attack.

The sight of Ethan's blood on Rafe's hands makes me nauseous. Helpless, I continue to yell from above, begging them to stop, but neither man acknowledges me.

Once Ethan has gained some distance from Rafe, he brings one foot up in the air and then jumps up and kicks that foot out. There's a sound like the crack of a whip as Ethan's foot connects with the side of Rafe's head, which rocks back from the force.

Rafe looks over at Ethan, his face a mask of pure rage. He swings wildly, but Ethan is ready and karate chops Rafe in the neck.

As Rafe reels back, Ethan again lashes out with his foot. The kick solidly contacts Rafe's head. Rafe claps his hand over his wounded head and wavers, blinking in pain. Ethan's fist comes from the left and punches Rafe in the jaw. It's the last blow. Rafe slumps to the ground, unconscious.

69

"Ethan!" My shouts have no effect. Ethan is frozen, staring down at Rafe's still form. I try again. "Ethan, I'm up here."

Finally, he raises his head to the ceiling. "Tiffy?"

"I'm here. Help me down."

Since he's tall, it's easy for Ethan to stand on the chair and get me out. I hold onto the bag of diamonds. As he places me gently on the ground, he asks, "You okay? Are you hurt?" His hands travel over my body, sweeping my arms and legs, searching for injuries.

I bat him away impatiently. "I'm fine. Really."

Looking at Ethan like I'm seeing him for the first time, I question, "What was that?"

He blinks owlishly at me, swaying as a thin line of blood trickles down his face. "What was what?" he asks, his words sluggish.

I snap my fingers in front of Ethan's unfocused eyes. Maybe he has a concussion? "Ethan. How did you do that?" I point down at Rafe's incapacitated body.

He shakes his head, trying to clear it, and follows my finger. "Oh, that." His gaze sharpens. "I told you." He widens his eyes, slightly exasperated. "I have a black belt. I've studied mixed martial arts. You know, the *Karate Kid* stuff?"

Admiration bubbles in my chest and with it the full realization that Ethan's *here*.

He came for me. I'm not alone.

Awed, I shake my head. "I can't believe it. Can't believe you fought like that."

"Tiffy." Ethan steps to me and places his hands on my cheeks, bracketing my face with his touch. A quiet desperation vibrates through his lean frame, a trembling in his fingertips, the adrenaline-fueled aftermath of battling with Rafe.

No tremor in his voice, though. It's steely, filled with determination. "I haven't had a lot of things I could call mine. Medicine was my parents' and my brother's. Baseball, maybe, but I lost that. But you, you're *mine,* and I'll be damned if I'm going to lose you. Not today. Not to that guy." He points to Rafe on the ground. "I will fight anything, or anyone, that comes between us. Nothing could keep me away from you. *Nothing.*" His composure breaks, and he draws me into a bone-crushing hug. "I was *so* worried. When you didn't come back. I lost it."

Pressed against his solid body, I rush to explain, "I wasn't running away. I swear. I—"

"Of course you weren't," he interrupts. "That didn't even cross my mind."

"It didn't?" I peer up at him.

"No. I know you. You keep your promises." He pulls me tighter, holding onto me like he's unmoored and I'm his anchor, the only thing tethering him to this reality where he got to me in time. Where I'm safe.

"What's going on? Who's this guy?" He doesn't let go, addressing all his questions to the top of my head.

Here it is.

The moment I've been dreading. He's been honest with me, and all I've given him in return are lies and secrets. I can't blame him when he walks away, but even if his abandonment is warranted I'll never get over it. Losing Ethan will wreck me. Shatter my heart into so many jagged pieces that I won't ever put it back together again.

Throat tight with unshed tears, I whisper, "You're going to hate me."

Ethan squeezes me even tighter. "Impossible." He pulls back from our embrace. Tilting my chin up with his hand, he forces me to meet his eyes. "I love you, Tiffy. I think I've loved you from the moment I first saw you glaring at me in that auditorium. Nothing can change that."

Ethan leans down and kisses me, long and slow. The world narrows down to this single sensation, the feeling of his lips pressed to mine. The brush of his tongue, the soft exhale of his breath. It awakens a firestorm of love within me. Hot tears break free at his touch and trickle down to mingle with our lips. He tenderly kisses each one away, and hope blossoms in my heart. Is there a chance, I wonder, however small, that he might still love me after he knows the truth? Can I be redeemed?

I'm lost in that thought when I suddenly remember the explosives. I push out of his arms, frantic. "Ethan! We need to get out of here. They're going to implode this building tonight!"

"What?" His eyes fly wide in disbelief.

"Yes. We need to leave right now!" I grip his upper arm tight, squeezing for emphasis.

"Okay." Ethan pauses and gestures at an unconscious Rafe. "Just one thing. What should we do with him?"

70

Together, we stare down at Rafe. He hasn't moved, not a single twitch.

"I'll call the police." Ethan reaches into his back pocket to retrieve his cell phone.

I still his movement with my hand. "Wait." Frozen in place, I lift my fingers to my forehead, which I rub, thinking hard.

"What? He kidnapped you," he insists.

But Ethan doesn't understand. He didn't grow up the way I did. He doesn't know the complicated web of history and loyalty I'm struggling with. So many memories flash before me. Rafe rescuing me at school and bloodying his knuckles for me. Rafe walking Shelly and me to our car each night. Rafe in a tuxedo, wanting so badly to fit in, to belong for just once in his life. To have a future where he's not the bad guy.

"Put your phone away," I say, quiet but firm.

The look Ethan sends me is incredulous, but he does as I request. I love him even more for that. For the trust and respect he has always given me, all the way back to the first day we met.

"Help me wake him up." I can see it's hard for Ethan. He's still keyed-up and angry from the fight. The need to protect me is radiating out of him.

Not too gently, he shoves his toe into Rafe's ribs and pushes, rolling Rafe back and forth with his foot.

"Hey, get up." Ethan's voice is gruff.

I join him, urging, "Rafe, wake up."

When Ethan looks over at me sharply, I ask, "What?"

"Rafe? You used to cry out that name when you had nightmares. I was so jealous, hearing another man's name from your lips. This is him?" Ethan pushes his toe even more aggressively into Rafe's ribs, almost kicking him.

I nod, not taking my eyes off Rafe, who stirs with a quiet groan. When Rafe wakes, he sees Ethan standing over him. He sits up and scrambles backward, putting distance between them. Rafe's gaze bounces suspiciously between Ethan and me.

Rafe notices the plastic bag at my feet. "You found them? The diamonds?" He stares greedily.

I step in front of the gemstones, partially blocking them from his view. "They aren't yours, Rafe."

His face darkens with anger. "That's not fair. You wouldn't know about them if I hadn't told you. You can't have them."

"You're right," I say, agreeing. "I can't have them, and neither can you. We never should have taken them. It was wrong."

"What are you going to do? Return them? Johnny's dead, remember?" Rafe argues.

"Dead? Diamonds? Tiffy, what's going on?" The bewildered look in Ethan's eyes pierces my heart. But I can't have this conversation right now. Not here, surrounded by the worst horrors of my past.

"Oh, Tiffany," Rafe says spitefully. "Didn't you tell him? About how you made money from selling your body on the Strip while you were in high school? Did you forget to mention that little detail? Did you forget to tell him about me?"

"Stop it," Ethan growls and takes a menacing step toward Rafe, but not before I see the shadow of betrayal in his eyes.

"Ethan, it wasn't like that. He's making it sound worse than it was." I grab his arm, attempting to turn Ethan's gaze away from Rafe and back to me. I'm desperate to make him understand, but he won't look at me.

"Please, Ethan. Listen to me—"

"Ignore her," Rafe interrupts, his gaze locked on Ethan. "Listen to *me*. That bag she's got has diamonds in it. You give the bag to me, and we'll split them. There's plenty for both of us." His grin is as slippery as a snake.

Ethan glares at Rafe, his lip curled in disgust. "No deal."

The smile slides off Rafe's face, leaving rage behind. He refocuses on me. "Come on, Tiffany. Give me the diamonds. I need them more than you do."

"Yeah, and what are you going to do with them? Drugs? Guns? More lives ruined?" I shake my head, crossing my arms over my chest.

"Not this time," he protests, placing a hand over his heart. "I'm going straight. I swear it."

"That's what you said last time, yet here we are, right where you left me." I fling a hand out, sweeping it over the dirty, decrepit room. "You'll have to forgive me, Rafe, but your promises mean nothing," I sneer, decades-old anger and resentment stirring to life. "Besides, the diamonds belong to Stewart. He's the next of kin."

Rafe scoffs, "Why? They didn't belong to Johnny. He stole them or got them as payment for something illegal, so they don't belong to Stewart either." He gives me a dismissive glance. "Are you really so naïve to think Stewart would do something noble with them? Do you know what he's been up to since you've been gone?"

He's got me there. I don't know where Stewart is or what he's doing now. It's been too painful to check up on him. If my actions had ruined his life, I don't think I could have gone on.

"I can give them to charity." I kick the bag lightly, the stones inside clinking together. "Donate them anonymously. Let them do some good for once."

Rafe snorts. His tone drips with condescension. "Do you really think the government will let them keep the diamonds? Whoever you're giving them to? Something so obviously stolen. The FBI will take them away, and no one will ever see them again. They might end up used for all the things you're so opposed to. Guns. Drugs. Who knows?"

What am I going to do? I imagine the diamonds, but now, instead of seeing them as something beautiful, something to covet, I picture them bathed in blood. How did Johnny get them? What kind of suffering were they payment for? He sure didn't get them for selling Girl Scout cookies. Maybe it would be better if they didn't exist. Then no one—not Rafe or Stewart or even me—could use them for our own gain.

"No. You aren't getting the diamonds, Rafe. No one is." I turn to Ethan. "Can you watch him for a minute?"

He nods once, face stern.

I pick up the bag, loop it over my fingers, and hurry out into the hallway. A couple of turns later, I stand next to a box of explosives. It has a heavy lid on it, which I pry off with some effort. Terrified, I stare at the sticks of dynamite and clay-like explosive material inside. Wires run in a thick bundle through the middle. I have no idea their purpose beyond the fact that at least one of them must trigger the detonation.

There are no windows in this hallway. No way to tell if it's day or night. How much time has passed since I entered the Starlight? How many hours, or maybe minutes, until the hotel implodes? If they triggered the explosives right now, I would be dead within seconds. It's like staring down the barrel of a gun.

Just as I'd hoped, there's some extra space in the box. The bag of jewels is heavy in my hands. The weight of them is heavy in my mind, too. I'm about to cram the bag into the box when, at the last minute, I hesitate. The diamonds are cold and sharp-edged against my skin as I plunge my hands into them. I take a fistful in each hand and quickly shove the sparkling gemstones into my pockets. The rest stay in the bag, which I place into the explosives box. I doubt Rafe will be clever enough to search in here. After I fit the lid on tight, I rush back to the supply room. The scene is exactly as I left it, Rafe and Ethan glaring at each other with tension crackling between them. What lies did Rafe tell Ethan while I was gone?

When I touch Ethan's arm, he flinches away. I drop my hand, stung. Ethan turns a grim, flat gaze to me, and I almost don't recognize him. Have I already lost him? Pain, actual physical pain, slices into my chest. I'm sure it's my heart breaking.

After I pull in a deep breath, I address Ethan and Rafe, my gaze moving back and forth between them. "We need to leave before they light this place up."

Meeting Rafe's eyes, I ask him, "Are you coming or not?"

He looks at us warily. I can see that he's calculating his chances of overcoming Ethan. But Ethan's roundhouse kick must have beaten some sense into him because, eventually, he nods. Rafe stands and, frowning heavily, joins Ethan and me as we leave the room and walk through the twisting hallways.

Ethan and I are a few steps ahead of Rafe so we exit the Starlight first, bursting into the fading desert sunset. Eagerly, I swallow huge gulps of fresh air. When I turn back, Rafe has paused inside the doorway of the hotel, still surrounded by its cold shadows.

"Come on." I wave my hand, motioning him forward.

Eyes rolling like a wild animal, Rafe shakes his head. "I can't."

"Of course you can." I hold my hand out, begging him to take it.

"You don't understand. They'll kill me." He's backing up now, one slow step at a time, heading deeper into the Starlight.

I have a vision then, a burst of imagination, that the hotel has come alive. It's a monster, with its claws wrapped around Rafe, gouging his flesh and dragging him into its gaping maw, ready to devour him.

This is it, my chance to save him like I've always dreamed. I move toward Rafe, stretching out my hand. My next step is halted by Ethan, who has grabbed my other arm and is pulling me away.

"Please, Rafe. Come with us," I plead, desperate. If he goes back into that darkness, he could die.

"No." Rafe shakes his head, swinging it wildly from side to side. "I'm sorry, but I can't." He turns and flees back into the ruined hotel.

And just like that, he's gone.

The Starlight swallows him whole.

71

Ethan and I watch the Starlight implode from our hotel room at the Venetian. It had been dark when we found the rental car in the overgrown parking lot, too late to book a flight out of Las Vegas. We decided to spend the night. He sits separated from me on the couch in the sunken sitting area of our room, with an ice pack on his knee, the bad one. Kicking Rafe has cost him. His knee is swollen and bruised. Every time I look at it, guilt twists, turning sour in my stomach.

I tried to talk to him on the drive over, had started to tell my story, but Ethan said he didn't want to discuss it, not yet. Now, we aren't talking at all, and the silence is killing me. I keep glancing at him out of the corner of my eye, and I don't like what I see. His face is devoid of emotion, an empty blank mask. I'm certain there are thoughts behind those dull eyes. He must have so many questions, but he's keeping them to himself. Or, even worse, maybe he doesn't want to hear my explanations. Maybe now that he's seen the *real* me, he no longer cares.

The TV announcer is talking in a loud, excited voice. I focus on the television to distract myself and see that Rafe was right. A program is airing all about the Starlight's history and demolition. Three television stations are offering live coverage, each broadcasting from a different angle.

The Starlight is across the street and down a block. If I press my face against the window in our room, I can see the edge of it and the enormous crowd of people gathered in front of the doomed hotel. They roar with anticipation so loud that we can hear them through both the windows of our room and the TV. It's like having surround sound stereo, the cheers echoing all around.

To me, the crowd seems bloodthirsty. Their applause makes me recall movies about ancient Rome when the spectators would clap gleefully right before a gladiator ran another through with his sword. I almost hate them, all these nameless strangers so eager to watch the past disappear. What dark thing is inside us, I wonder, that makes us drawn to destruction? Why do we yell louder when we watch something unravel in minutes than when we watch something take years to build?

Patriotic music plays over loudspeakers as the grand finale of fireworks goes off behind the Starlight. Each bang of fireworks sounds like a gunshot.

Please let Rafe be gone from there. Let him be safe.

Rafe must have gotten out by now. He isn't stupid. Surely, he understood the danger. I haven't forgiven him for how he abducted me and brought me to Las Vegas, but that doesn't mean I want him to die. Did Rafe find the diamonds? I think it's unlikely, but who knows? He was desperate, which made him unpredictable.

A laser countdown is projected on the side of the old hotel and casino.

The crowd chants along.

5, 4, 3, 2, 1.

The explosives are lit. A bright spark begins in the center and, almost too quick for my eyes to follow, rushes to the outer edges of the old building. A bang sounds, so loud and booming that the windows of our hotel room rattle violently.

The Starlight collapses in on itself, a house of cards caught in a breeze. It goes down. A lifetime of memories disappears in a matter of seconds. A huge plume of gray dust rises billowing out of the ruined structure. The debris spreads out farther than the event planners had anticipated. Onlookers who are closest to the spectacle get caught in the storm. They run from it, gagging and choking.

The diamonds are gone forever. I picture them ground into a fine dust by the explosion. Thrown up into the atmosphere to glitter in the sky alongside the stars. When it's all over, I'm surprised to find that my cheeks are wet. Even though I have mostly terrible memories from the hotel, I didn't enjoy watching it crumble. It's just one more thing from my past that's died.

With a click of the remote, Ethan turns off the TV. The room is dim without its flickering light. The blare of the television is gone, leaving behind an uncomfortable silence.

"What…" I trail off, chasing the train of my thoughts. There are things I need to ask him. Things I need to tell him. "I have so many questions. How did you find me?" I still can't wrap my mind around it. Seeing Ethan at the Starlight had been surreal.

He won't meet my eye as he answers, "Simple. You put your username and password on my phone when you downloaded the Disney app. My phone saved it. I used that to log into your email account, where I saw the plane tickets you bought to come here."

"But how did you know about the Starlight?"

"You mentioned it once, remember? Plus, when you went missing, I asked around, trying to find anyone who had seen you. Eventually, a worker at the hotel said a pretty redhead was arguing with a dude three times her size. With that description, I knew it was you."

The hotel worker who had been clearing off the breakfast buffet. It must have been him.

Ethan's still talking. "He heard something about a place that started with the word star. I put two and two together."

"Ethan," I begin. "I want to explain about what Rafe said. About everything."

Dropping his head into his hands, Ethan sighs wearily. "I'm not sure I'm ready to hear it."

"Well, too bad, because I have to tell you." So I do. I tell him all about my childhood, about my mom, Brandi, Shelly, Mr. Chen, and Rafe. I tell him about myself. The good and the bad. When I was strong and the many times I was weak. It hurts to talk about it all. Several times I need to stop because I'm crying.

Even my tears don't bring Ethan over to my side.

When my tale is done, he says, "I don't know, Tiffany. I don't know what to say." He sounds exhausted. His fingers stroke the scar in his eyebrow, rubbing it so hard the skin reddens.

The use of my full name is a pickax to my heart. "Please, Ethan. I know it's bad. At the time, I couldn't see another way out."

"It's not that. It's not the photos on the Strip or even the robbery. I understand all of that. You were a child placed in an impossible situation." His voice has been a monotone, but now it rises. "The part I don't get is how you never told *me* any of this. All the time I was talking to you, telling you about my family, my past. You said nothing. I told you things I've never spoken aloud before. *Never.* And you just sat there, holding all these secrets. You didn't trust me enough to let me in. *That's* what I can't understand."

My tears fall freely. With a trembling hand, I dash them away. "I should have told you. I'm sorry. So sorry I didn't. Please." I can't breathe. This can't be happening. It's another nightmare.

Ethan stands and goes to stare out the window into the night. The many lights of the Las Vegas Strip twinkle through the sheer curtains. It maddens me to see those lights. How dare they shine when my world is going dark?

Without looking away from the window, he says, "Let's go to bed. It's late. We can talk about it in the morning."

He walks past me to the bathroom, giving me a wide berth. The click of the lock when he closes the door so he can brush his teeth is as loud as the Starlight's explosion. That's when I know he's water slipping through my fingers, the ocean pulling away from the shore, the sun running from the moon.

I get it. If I'm being honest and our roles were reversed, would I be able to forgive him? I'm not sure I could. I would feel too misled, too betrayed. My temper and ego would stand between us, an enormous wall too high to climb. Is it really fair for me to expect Ethan to look past all my omissions when I wouldn't be able to do the same?

We'll talk about it in the morning.

Yeah, right.

Liar.

I heard it—the finality in his voice. He's already gone, and I'll never get him back. Because of my foolish insecurities and mistruths, I've lost Ethan. The worst part is I didn't even get to tell him I love him.

72

We lay in bed, with our backs to each other. It's been hours, but I can't sleep. Ethan's awake too, I can tell. We've spent so much time together in close quarters that I'm attuned to his breathing. How it deepens and evens out when he drifts off. I haven't heard that tonight. In the darkness, he shifts restlessly. The sheets rustle as they slide over his body. He exhales. Kicks his legs under the covers, pulls the covers up, then pushes them down.

I hold still, paralyzed by the images that flash through my mind. Rafe. Diamonds. The Starlight as it fell. The one that replays the most is the split second of betrayal that crossed Ethan's face when he realized that I hadn't been honest with him. That wounded look is keeping me up. I can't stand it, knowing I was the one to make him feel that pain.

I'm crying again, silently. It reminds me of all the times at Mr. Chen's when I sobbed in bed next to my mother. How I learned to swallow the sound of my tears so I wouldn't disturb her.

Somehow, Ethan hears me. The bed shakes as he rolls over so he's facing my shuddering back. "Don't cry, Tiffy. Please, don't cry." His whisper is so soft that for a moment I think it's my imagination. Then I realize he's talking to me. When he says my special nickname, it hurts so bad I whimper.

Strong arms slide under my neck and around my shoulder. Ethan pulls me back to him, reeling me into his chest. Spooning me. He presses me close and leans his cheek against my head.

"Shhh," he soothes.

"I'm sorry. So sorry." I'm choking on my tears, drowning in them.

He nestles closer, wrapping his leg around mine. "I'm sorry, too," he breathes into my ear. I break free and roll over to face him. His arms find their place around me again. I stare into his amber eyes, hoping he can see that my regret is sincere.

"I should have told you," I confide in a whisper. "I was just so scared."

"It's okay." He brushes my hair off my cheek and tucks it behind my ear, the gesture reminding me of happier times.

"No, it's not. I would be devastated if you did that to me." My fingers curl into fists that lie useless against his collarbones.

Ethan cups my cheek, brushing his thumbs lightly under my puffy eyes. "It's just that I want to know all of you, every little thing. I had hoped you would tell me your secrets not because you *had* to, but because you *wanted* to. When I found out that you hadn't, it hurt."

"I wanted to tell you, but I thought if you knew I would lose you." My voice trembles as my hands unfurl and press against his chest, seeking the solace of his heartbeat.

"You won't lose me. Remember? You're stuck with me." He gives me a small smile, tinged with sadness. "I should be the one apologizing, Tiffy. You needed me tonight, but I've been too busy nursing my upset feelings. I forgot that you have wounds that need healing too."

I shake my head, unable to believe I'm forgiven.

He leans forward and places a soft kiss on my forehead. "You've accepted me for who I am, all the good and all the bad. Now, let me do the same for you."

I gather my courage. "I love you, Ethan. So, so much."

Of all his many smiles, this is the biggest, the most brilliant.

"You know," he says, his smile fading into a serious look, "sometimes good people do bad things. I think the person you need forgiveness from the most isn't me. I think it's *you*. You need to forgive yourself."

His words make me cry even harder because he's right. All the self-loathing. All the blame I've carried. It's held me back from the life I want. A life full of love and acceptance. The same emotions I see in Ethan's eyes. His love for me shines there, so brightly. Sniffling, I nod my head, agreeing with him.

"I love you, Tiffy. Nothing can change that." He bends his lips to mine. The kiss starts out slowly but builds to red-hot quickly. Hands on the nape of my neck, Ethan crushes his mouth against me. It's demanding, territorial. All his earlier fear pours into me, like he needs this physical connection to verify that I really am here with him. That he didn't lose me to Rafe or to the explosion. He needs the reassurance of my mouth, my touch. My body answers Ethan's need. I give myself up to him, returning his kiss with equal fervor. We kiss for what seems like forever, until I break off the motion with a yawn.

"You're tired." He points at my yawn, which I try to hide behind my hand.

"I'm fine." I kiss him again, relishing the sensation.

Ethan ends the kiss, gently pulling away. "Time for bed." He moves my head onto his shoulder and slings a leg over my thigh, tucking my body into his.

I'm still protesting weakly, but I'm too sleepy to put any weight behind my words. The sheets are cool, and Ethan's body is warm.

An idea has been simmering in my mind. "Ethan?"

"Hmm?" he asks sleepily.

"Can we stay here one more day? There's something I need to do."

His hands are in my hair, slowly running his fingers through the length of it. "Sure."

Exhausted, we drift off together. My dreams feature an always smiling man with warm amber eyes. Happy dreams, full of abstract colors and ideas I won't remember in the morning.

73

It isn't hard to locate Stewart. A few minutes on Google and I learn he's still at the Luxor, only now he's risen to become the Chief Director of Operations, which is a fancy way of saying that he runs the whole casino. His professional title surprises me. I can't picture the awkward introvert I remember as the boss of so many people. That job would take an awful lot of handshaking and elbow-rubbing.

It takes a few calls, but eventually I get in touch with him. Our conversation on the phone is brief, just long enough to agree to meet at a local park at noon. I have no idea what to expect from him, so an open neutral meeting place seems like a good idea.

Plus, I've spent all morning arguing with Ethan. He wants to come with me to meet Stewart. After the encounter with Rafe, he's extra-protective of me. He hasn't let me out of his sight. Eventually, I compromised with Ethan. I'll meet Stewart in the park while Ethan waits for me in the car, but only if he can see me the entire time.

When we pull into the parking lot, my palms are sweating. I still haven't figured out what I'm going to say. In my mind, I've practiced multiple explanations for my past actions, but nothing seems quite right. How do you apologize to someone you haven't seen in over a decade? How do you justify deliberately hurting them?

Ethan turns the rental car off, and we sit together in silence, listening to the ticking sound of the engine as it cools. It's a cloudless fall day, the wind brisk and the trees bare. The sun is a white orb high in the sky, but today it provides little warmth. I pull the cardigan sweater that I bought in the hotel gift shop tighter around my chest.

Hands still on the steering wheel, Ethan asks, "Are you ready?"

"Yes. I mean no…but yes."

A sleek black sedan with heavily tinted windows glides into the lot across from us. A burly man in a dark suit gets out of the driver's seat. There's a gleam as the sunlight hits a small earpiece made of clear plastic with a cord running down his neck, like something a Secret Service agent would wear.

The driver walks around the car to the back door and opens it. A thin man steps out, and I recognize him as Stewart, although he's ditched the jeans and white tennis shoes for a well-tailored dark gray suit and expensive-looking leather dress shoes.

"I can come with you," Ethan offers again.

I frown and shake my head. "No. I want to do this alone. I need to talk to him, just me. No distractions."

Looking like he wants to argue but knows better, Ethan leans across the center console of the car and gives me a firm kiss.

"Be careful," he warns as he pulls away. "I'm here if you need me."

When I step out of the car, Stewart looks past me into the car at Ethan. He's seen the kiss, but his face remains impassive.

"Stewart—" I begin before he cuts me off.

"Let's go talk over there." Stewart juts his chin toward a picnic table under a pergola. It's a short distance away.

"Okay." We don't speak as we walk over to the table. The silence is thick and heavy with tension. I nervously wipe my hands along the front of my pants as I sit down. The metal bench is cold beneath me with dried-up gum crusted under its edges.

Marshaling my courage, I say, "Thanks for meeting me here."

There are no cracks in Stewart's poker face. "I was surprised to hear from you, obviously. It made me curious to find out why you wanted to get together."

I pause, wondering when Stewart changed. His demeanor is different now, so remote and calculating. Not a single stutter. Did he begin this transformation the day I lied to him, the day his father died? How much am I responsible for the man I see before me today?

I reach into my pocket and take out a Ziploc bag full of diamonds. Two fistfuls of them, to be exact. I place the bag on the table and shove it at Stewart.

He barely glances at the gems, which shimmer with their own internal fire. "What're those?"

"A peace offering." It may have been the wrong thing to do, but I couldn't come to him empty-handed. I'm hoping he'll see the diamonds as a symbolic gesture of good faith.

No response from him.

"You're pretty calm for someone who just got a bunch of priceless jewels," I observe with surprise. Maybe I was fooling myself, but I thought my gift would evoke some kind of emotion.

"I run a casino, Tiffany. Bags of gemstones aren't uncommon in my business," he says dryly.

Oh. Well, I guess I hadn't thought of that.

"What do you want?" Stewart's gaze narrows and his lips arch downward. His hand reaches out to sweep the bag off the table and into his lap. Guess he's keeping them.

"To talk to you. To say I'm sorry. I don't know what you figured out about that night at the masquerade party, but I lied to you and I regret it. What I did was unconscionable. You were my friend, and I betrayed your trust. I understand it won't help, but I think about it all the time. I've spent years beating myself up for what I did." The words tumble out, tripping over themselves in their rush to escape.

Stewart's eyes narrow even more. "Is that supposed to make me feel better? Knowing that you think about it? Well, I think about it too." Finally showing some emotion, his voice crackles with anger. "You hurt me, Tiffany. When you ran away, guess who had to pick up the pieces? I lost someone who I was starting to have feelings for at the same time I lost my father." He makes a face, like it pains him to admit that he had liked me.

His words skewer me. I know how lonely grief can be. He lost his parent and was left all alone, just like I was. Why didn't I see it at that time? If

I hadn't messed up, we could have helped each other through that terrible experience. I was a fool to lose that opportunity.

Stewart's still talking. "And I had to cover the tracks you stupidly left behind."

I had been right. Stewart had protected me, had done whatever he needed to do in order to hide my crime. No wonder the police never came. I swallow hard, realizing that if he hadn't intervened, my entire life could have turned out differently. All my dreams of becoming a doctor came true because of what he did.

"I appreciate that, Stewart. You have no idea how much. Everything in my life I owe to your shielding me from my own dumb, selfish mistakes. I'm sorry I put you in that position, but it was kind of you to help me. I didn't deserve it."

Tears threaten, but I won't yield to them. I don't want Stewart to believe I'm trying to manipulate him in any way. I've promised myself to be completely honest during this conversation. To throw away all the false masks I've worn over the years.

"You sure as heck didn't." An angry scowl dominates Stewart's features. "You could have asked me, you know. If you needed money, you could have told me and I would have helped."

"I know you would, but I couldn't do that. I didn't want to end up beholden to you. That would have been leading you on, which I was trying not to do." I shift on the uncomfortable bench.

"Agreeing to come to a party with me and wearing a pretty dress wasn't leading me on? If you were trying to avoid that, then you did a poor job of it." His clenched jaw ticks.

"You're right. I'm sorry." There's nothing else to say. I knew this would be a hard conversation, but a little part of me had hoped that Stewart would forgive me. I'm losing that hope now.

Mouth in a straight line, he stays silent, not accepting my apology. Again, I'm taken aback by the changes in Stewart. His face is stern, and his eye contact is direct. It makes me sad, missing the bashful sweet man I had known.

How we all have changed.

"Wait," I say, a thought occurring to me. "If you covered for me, then why did the guard try to stop us when we were leaving the Luxor?"

"They stopped everyone from the party. The police tried to retain all the guests for questioning because of the shooting. They wanted statements from the witnesses." *Oh yeah, I was still wearing my mask so the guard would have known I was from the party.* It all makes sense now. Stewart shoots me a look like he can't believe I didn't figure it out on my own, but how could I? Back then, I was too wrapped up in my guilt to think through all the possibilities.

Stewart's eyes shift to something behind me. I follow his gaze and see he's looking at the car where Ethan stares at us intently.

"Looks like you have a bodyguard with you today," he comments.

"No bodyguard. He's my," I pause, uncertain how to describe Ethan. We haven't had the "define our relationship" talk yet, but given the declaration of love he made yesterday I feel confident enough to say, "my boyfriend."

"He knows about the diamonds you just gave away?" He arches a brow and tilts his head, blinking at me owlishly.

"Yes, he does." I had told Ethan about my plan this morning, and he had agreed it was a good idea. It was a relief to be honest with him. I won't *ever* lie to him again.

"Besides, I'm pretty sure you have a much more professional bodyguard than I do." I wave toward Stewart's town car and the brawny man inside. "Is it always like that?" I ask him. "Do you always have a bodyguard with you now that you run the Luxor?"

His face is grim. "I usually have someone with me if I don't want to end up like my father." He sighs, and some of his anger seems to deflate as the air blows out of him. "It's a hard job running a casino. Always surrounded by people, but I'm still alone. Maybe it's better this way. I never was much good at making or keeping friends."

An urge to reassure Stewart that I'm his friend comes over me, but I hold my tongue. That would be overstepping. As much as I want him to realize he's not alone, I understand I gave away our friendship when I accepted the invitation to that party. Still, Ethan has shown me how persistence and patience can thaw even the most frozen heart. Hopefully, there's still a chance with Stewart.

"Look," I begin. I brace for rejection but plow ahead anyway. "I don't deserve it. You have every right to say no, but would it be all right if I emailed you sometimes? Maybe called you just to see how you're doing? You may not believe me, but I really counted you as my friend."

Lips pursed, Stewart contemplates my offer. "What about your boyfriend? Wouldn't that bother him?"

Glancing again at Ethan, I send him a tight smile to reassure him that I'm okay. "He's not like that. He trusts me."

Stewart stares at an empty space over my head, his lips tight in a frown. "I don't know about being friends again. I'm not sure I can do that with you. Not sure I want to."

Even though I'm expecting it, hearing his words stings. I look down at the mottled brown-green grass under my feet. "I understand."

A plane drones overhead, the only sound between us.

Finally, Stewart stands up. He takes a quick breath. "I'll think about it. That's the best I can do."

Wind stirs the leaves by our feet, and I shiver. I gather my sweater tight and button it up. As we walk back to the parking lot, I tell him, "That's all I'm asking for." I'm grateful for even that small glimmer of hope. I truly want to mend our relationship.

It's time to make friends again.

74

PRESENT, COLUMBUS, OHIO

"Hurry up, Tiffy, or we'll be late," calls Ethan from the living room.

With only a towel wrapped around me, I stand in my closet, flipping through hangers. I'm trying to decide between the black dress or the green one. I shoot off a quick text to Melanie.

> *Tiffany: What are you wearing tonight?*
>
> *Melanie: My blue jumper. U?*
>
> *Tiffany: Can't decide between my green or black dress.*

I send her a photo of each one.

> *Melanie: The green. It brings out your eyes. Ethan will be all Ooh La La when he sees you.*
>
> *Tiffany: Melanie!*
>
> *Melanie: What? It's true! I see the way he looks at you.*
>
> *Melanie: Hey, thanks again for helping me pick out Flooffy the Cat. She's the best, but she keeps scratching the furniture…and me. Is that normal?*

Tiffany: She's a kitten, so yeah. Totally normal. Also, still can't believe you named her Flooffy.

Melanie: Why? What's wrong with Flooffy?? I just love her so much, and I want to cuddle but her claws are tiny razors!

Tiffany: Tomorrow we'll go to the pet store and get a scratching post.

Melanie: Okay. Thanks. See U soon.

Tiffany: See you.

Back in my bedroom, as I slide the green dress up and over my hips, my eyes land on my favorite picture. It's a photo of Ethan and me from Disney World. We're standing in front of Cinderella's castle. Ethan had surprised me, grabbing me and dipping me backward with a kiss just as the cast member had taken the shot. In the picture, we're laughing even as our lips touch.

Those last two days at the medical conference in Orlando had been magical. With all the Las Vegas drama behind us, we finally had time to embrace our new relationship. It had been all about holding hands, laughing, and kissing.

Next to the picture is my Resident of the Month award. I received it when I got back from Orlando. Dr. Washburn said it was my reward for all the good work I had done, both in Cleveland and at the conference in Florida. As a surprise, Ethan had it framed for me. At one point in my life, that certificate had meant everything to me. Even though I'm grateful I got it, I have so much more to be thankful for now.

"Tiffy, you ready?" Ethan walks into my bedroom. He's so handsome, all tall and masculine. His scent, soap and mint, fills my nose as he moves closer. It's familiar and comforting, putting me at ease.

"Almost." I turn my back to him. "Can you help me pull up the zipper?" I gather my hair to the side so it won't get caught.

He puts his mouth on my shoulder and gives it a playful nip. "I'd rather kiss you." His voice is deep and husky in my ear.

The corners of my mouth tug upward. "Weren't you the one telling me to hurry?"

"Maybe I was wrong." Ethan's mouth moves to the crook of my neck, which he kisses softly. "Maybe we should slow down rather than hurry up. We can be late, can't we?"

Breathless from his touch, I struggle to concentrate. "No. You were right. Melanie and her boyfriend will be waiting. They won't keep going on double dates with us if we're always late."

"Fine." There's the sound of the zipper being pulled up. I let my hair drop to hang in long shiny waves. I turn to a pouting Ethan and place my hands on his shoulders. Standing on my tiptoes, I press my lips to his.

"Aren't you going to see Melanie tomorrow, anyway? When you get your nails done?" he asks plaintively.

"Yes. We're getting manicures with Natalie." It makes me happy, thinking about how much fun it will be to spend time with my girlfriends at the nail salon. Since I got back from Florida, I've been hanging out with Melanie and her best friend, Natalie. They've been wonderful, including me in all their plans.

"That doesn't excuse us for being late." Standing on one leg at a time, I put on my black strappy heels. That done, I straighten the hem of my dress and glance up to find Ethan's admiring gaze roving over my body. It makes me catch my breath, the way his amber eyes light up on me.

"You're gorgeous." He runs his hand down my bare arm, leaving goosebumps behind. "Don't worry. We won't be late, my little rule follower." A lopsided smirk, amusement dancing in his expression.

I feel a swell of love for him, this handsome, smart, and loyal man. He's so perfectly perfect for me. With my heels on, I don't have to reach as far to give him a deep kiss. Softly, I confess. "I love you." Another heart-melting kiss. "Have I told you recently that I'm glad you're here with me?"

Ethan grins crookedly. "It's like I'm always telling you. You're stuck with me."

Epilogue

It's been a busy day in the hospital, but things are finally winding down when the lead tech, Amy, walks into my office.

"Dr. Hart?" she says, waiting patiently for me to finish the case I'm working on.

Done, I spin my chair around to face her. I glance at the other chair in the room. It's empty. Ethan's at the other hospital across town today, and I miss him.

"What can I do for you, Amy?"

"There's a patient here for you, Dr. Hart. He asked for you specifically."

My eyebrows rise. It's unusual in radiology to have patients request a specific doctor. "Okay. Where is he?" I push out of my chair and pull on my long white coat, its pockets heavy with my stethoscope and pens.

Amy follows me out into the hallway. "I had him stay in the lobby. Our waiting room is still pretty full. I swear the nice summer weather has made every single person go outside and break a bone today."

I agree. It's been nonstop X-rays for fractured bones for the past couple of hours.

"Anyway," continues Amy, "you won't be able to miss this guy. He's tall, dark, and handsome." She winks at me. "I wouldn't mind if he requested to see me, that's for sure."

Rolling my eyes at her, I head for the hospital lobby. My curiosity has been piqued. Once I pass the coffee cart, I spot him. A man with eyes like emeralds stands by the sliding lobby doors.

Rafe.

I freeze, my heart pounding. I have thought about him so many times, wondering if he got out of the Starlight in time. Seeing him here, whole and unharmed, brings a sense of relief. It's quickly followed by apprehension. What does he want? Money? Revenge?

Expressionless, Rafe watches me cross the room.

"What are you doing here?" I ask when I reach him.

Now that I'm up close, I see that he looks different from the last time I saw him. He's gained some weight. The hollows of his cheeks and under his eyes are less pronounced. Clean-shaven, he has on a newish-looking button-down shirt and a nice pair of jeans. His hair is shorter than before. Most importantly, his green eyes are warm as he regards me.

Still uncertain of his motives, I ask, "Do you…need something?" Given that I'm not sensing Rafe's usual hostility, I wonder even more why he's here.

Maybe something's wrong. Is he sick and needs my help? Is it about Shelly? All the questions flood my mind at once. "Are you okay?"

Rafe's face is relaxed, and his smile is the warmest I've ever seen. "Actually, I'm better than okay. I've made…some changes since the last time I saw you, and things are good now."

"What are you doing here?" My forehead creases.

He gestures to a pair of upholstered chairs in the corner of the room. Following his lead, I sit next to him. "There's something I've been meaning to tell you. Something that's bothered me for a long time." He pauses, running his hand over the back of his neck. "It's about the night of the party. I was talking to Johnny the Shark. I didn't really know him well. We'd only worked a couple of jobs together before he died." Rafe checks to make sure I'm listening. "He must have seen us together because he asked me about you, Tiffany."

"He did? He asked about me?" I point to myself.

"Yeah. He wanted to know about you and your mom. I didn't know why he was so interested. I still don't totally understand, but here's where it gets weird. Johnny looked scared, the only time in my life I saw that man frightened. Even when he got shot later, he didn't look like that. Only when he talked about you."

"Why?" I purse my lips, thinking back to that night. Johnny *had* given me a strange look when I first met him. He had stared at my dress with an odd expression, almost like recognition, but he didn't seem frightened. More like he was perplexed. "Surely, he wasn't scared of *me*?"

"No." A brief shake of his head. "He mentioned your dad."

"My dad? My dad is dead." I cross my leg over my knee and lean forward, listening intently.

"You sure? Because Johnny didn't seem to think so." Rafe looks around suspiciously and lowers his voice. "I can't remember the exact words, but Johnny said something about if your dad ever found out where you were, he would burn down the world to get to you. That's when he looked scared."

"I don't understand. What does it mean?" I ask helplessly.

Rafe frowns. "I honestly don't know, but the way he said it stood out to me. I made myself remember all the details so I could tell you." His hand rubs the back of his neck again. "I had a bad feeling about it. I've always thought I should warn you."

Squeezing my eyes shut, I shake my head. "You came all this way just to tell me that?"

"Basically. I felt like I owed you…you know, for the last time I saw you." Rafe looks away.

"Oh, you mean the time you kidnapped me, blackmailed me, and forced me into an abandoned building that was about to be blown to smithereens? That last time?" I can't keep the sarcasm from my voice.

Rafe has the decency to look ashamed. "Yeah, that last time."

I'm silent, trying to puzzle out what he's revealed. If only my mom was still alive to answer the questions about my dad, but, as usual, I'm on my own. Well, not totally on my own, because I have Ethan now and he'll help me find any answers I need. I swallow down the anxiety that Rafe's revelation has given me and lower my voice. "You know what's weird?"

"What?"

"The money we stole from Johnny wasn't enough for all my mom's medical bills. When I tried later to pay the rest, the hospital told me the debt was settled. Someone paid the rest of it. I asked them who, but they looked and there was no record. It was like all that data had been wiped clean. At the time, I thought maybe it was Stewart." I sigh, frustrated by all these unanswered questions. "Could that have anything to do with my dad?"

"Don't know. It makes me wonder." Rafe leans back in his chair, his bulky frame filling it completely. "We may never know. If someone had the power to erase the payment records, then they obviously don't want you to find them."

Staring at my hands clasped in my lap, I ponder what this all means. He stands, towering over me. "I'd better take off. I've got a flight to catch."

"Where are you going?" I tilt my head, curious.

"Someplace warm." He's being deliberately vague, but I don't blame him. Probably better for me not to know.

"Here." He hands me a scrap of paper with some numbers scribbled on it. "This is my phone number. If you ever need anything, just call." Rafe laughs, the sound almost lighthearted. "Not that you're likely to need me, since your boyfriend fights like a ninja." He rubs the side of his head. "I can still feel where he kicked me."

"Sorry about that, but you did kind of bring it on yourself." I stand and pat him on the shoulder.

He meets my eyes, his gaze steady. "I'm glad you have someone who will fight for you. We should all have someone who loves us that much."

Without thinking, I hug Rafe, rising onto my toes and throwing my arms lightly around his waist. He goes stiff for a second and then relaxes, his arms winding around my shoulders. "Good-bye, Tiffany." He squeezes gently before releasing me. "Take care of yourself."

"Bye, Rafe." I take a step back and watch as he walks away. The automatic doors open and close behind him, and I wonder if I'll ever see him or Shelly again.

My phone buzzes in my coat pocket, startling me. I put it on vibrate earlier when I was with a patient. Fishing it out, I see that Ethan's name flashes on the screen.

"Hey. You'll never believe who I just saw," I tell him as soon as I accept the call.

Ethan's voice rumbling in my ear makes me smile. That's all it takes, just the sound of his voice. "Who? Tell me. I'm on my way to pick you up. How do you feel about me making you dinner tonight?"

A glance at my watch shows my shift is over. "I feel all kinds of good about you making me dinner. I'll tell you about my surprise visitor then."

"Sounds good. I don't have anything for dessert, though," he warns.

With a wicked smile, I tap into my now-perfected flirt and purr into the phone. "Sure you do—me."

"Mmm," Ethan murmurs appreciatively. "My favorite. Be there in a minute. Oh, and Tiffy?"

"Yes?" I head back to my office to gather my things.

"I love you," says Ethan.

"Love you, too."

The End

BONUS EPILOGUE!!

Hello, dear reader, I'm sure right now you're wondering, "But what about Fred The Cat? What does he think about Tiffany and Ethan's relationship?" What?? You weren't thinking about that? *Huh.*

Well, click this link anyway to read a hysterical bonus epilogue from Fred The Cat's point of view and join my newsletter where I give you FREE chapters of my upcoming novels, updates, giveaways, and more.

HTTPS://TINYURL.COM/FRED-THE-CAT-BONUS

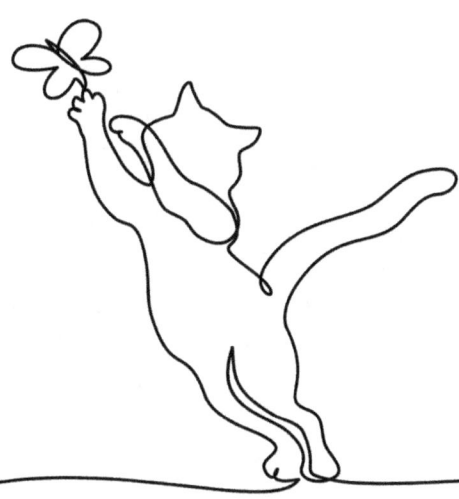

THANKS FOR READING!

Can I please ask you, dear reader, for a BIG favor? If you enjoyed this book, pretty please leave a review.

I know that your time is precious, but reviews are what make or break an author's career. They influence everything from reaching new readers to training Amazon's algorithms to put this book on the top of the page when you search for it.

I personally read every review, and your feedback helps me write the books YOU want to read. We are in this together, you and I.

So, thank you a million times over for reading this book and for leaving a review. You are literally making my dreams come true.

XOXO, Melissa

Here's the link and QR code to review.

HTTPS://TINYURL.COM/REVIEWDRHARTSWEET

DO YOU LIKE GAMES?

Me, too!

I'm a BIG Swiftie. In this story, I have hidden
10 Taylor Swift song lyrics and titles.

Can you find one or more of them?

Email me if you do!
hello@melissadymondauthor.com

I have some special prizes that I'm ONLY sharing
with winners of this challenge, so email me your answer and,
if you get it right, I'll send you the prize! Let's play!

BONUS: HOLIDAY STAR FREE FIRST CHAPTER

Have you read this celebrity romance yet? Get it now!

HTTPS://TINYURL.COM/HOLIDAYSTARSWEET

ONE house.
ONE doctor.
ONE movie star.
What could go wrong?
It's not like they're going to fall in love, right?

PROLOGUE

"OHMYGOD! There he is," Jenny whispers in a high-pitched squeal, her hand on my arm, nails digging into my skin. I don't even bother to lift my gaze from my plate. I know who she's referring to. *Caleb Lawson.* He's the *only* thing she's been talking about tonight.

"I can't believe he's your cousin now." She rips a dinner roll in half, smears it with butter, and shoves it into her mouth, all without taking her eyes off the man across the room.

"He's *not* my cousin." I'm exasperated because we've had this conversation at least a dozen times. She's mostly kidding, but honestly, I'm tired of her bringing it up. "He's the son of my stepfather's sister."

My *new* stepfather.

I search through the crowded ballroom until I find my mother in her long white dress. She's beautiful, flowers woven into her hair, diamond earrings, an early wedding gift from her husband, dangling from her ears. Talking with some distant relatives, she waves her expressive hands.

As I watch, my new stepdad, Seth, comes up behind her. He winds an arm around her waist and joins the conversation. Mom leans into him, relaxing into that embrace like it's the most natural thing. She's happy today, on her wedding day.

I'm happy for her, too.

I'm just sad for me.

Which is a bad feeling, a selfish one. My dad passed away almost nine years ago, and Mom had waited a *long* time before she dated. She waited until my older brother and I had moved out and my younger brother was a senior in high school, applying for college.

Once she finally started dating, she met Seth pretty quickly. When Mom knew she could have a future with him, she spoke to each of us individually, asking for our permission before they got serious.

It shouldn't bother me when Seth takes her hand and leads her out onto the dance floor. She deserves it, to be loved once again. I know this. I believe it wholeheartedly.

But, much to my dismay, it does bother me. Because all I can see is my father spinning her around our living room, dancing in the colorful glow of the Christmas tree. The sound of their laughter and how they stared into each other's eyes as if no one else existed.

I have to remind myself *that* is a memory, and *this* is reality.

Looking away from the dance floor, I take in the understated cream-colored ballroom. Simple flower arrangements of white roses and lilies sit on tables that are ringed by slip-covered chairs. Crystal chandeliers cast a warm glow over the guests as they chat and mingle.

Out of the window, it's a picture-perfect Santa Monica day. The Pacific

Ocean glistens with white-capped waves. Surfers balance, arms outstretched, only to topple into the water as the swell they ride crashes into the sand.

Mom lets out a tinkling laugh, drawing my attention back to her. I watch as Seth twirls her around the dance floor, causing her white wedding dress to flare out into a bell shape.

I have a dress like that, too. It's in a garment bag, shoved deep into the back of my closet. Never worn.

"Do you think it's possible to be equal parts happy and sad at the same time?" I ask Jenny, fiddling with the place card in front of me. It has my name on it, in swooping cursive script.

Dr. Gwen Wright.

Before Jenny can answer, my older brother, Brandon, comes over. "You're up," he tells me. I rise and follow him to the raised dais in the center of the room, where a microphone sits on a stand, waiting for me.

Mom and Seth have finished their dance and taken their seats at the long, narrow table reserved for the wedding party. I glance over, and Mom gives me an encouraging smile.

Anxious, I rearrange the wide skirts of my lacy, blue bridesmaid dress. Next to me, Brandon taps a fork against a crystal goblet. The loud ringing sound echoes through the room, drawing everyone's attention. Brandon hands me the microphone and takes a step back, leaving me alone in the spotlight, a place that feels unfamiliar. Insecurity batters at me, chipping away at the confidence I've built over the years.

When I look into the crowd, my gaze snags on my younger brother Teddy, who sits two tables down with his suit jacket off and his tie askew. He gives me a cheesy thumbs up, trying to bolster my spirits. I send a shaky smile back.

After I clear my throat, I say, "Hello, everyone." The microphone lets out a high-pitched hiss of feedback. I readjust it and begin again, sounding unnaturally loud. "I'm Gwen, the daughter of the bride and also the maid of honor. Thank you all for joining my family and me today as we celebrate the marriage of my mother, Melinda, and Seth.

"As most of you already know, I have the best mother in the world. She puts her children first. Whether it was staying up late to help us finish a project for school or cuddling with us on the couch when we were sick, Mom was always there for us."

I pause, swallowing down the knot in my throat, anxious about the next part. I hadn't been sure how to address my father's death from colon cancer in this toast. If I should ignore it because it's too morbid or mention it as a way to honor him and to acknowledge all the hardships my family went through after he died. In the end, I included him. I still think of my dad every day and to leave him out had felt like a betrayal.

"After my father passed away, I worried that as much as she cared for us, my mom also needed someone to care for her. When she met Seth and fell in love with him, I knew I didn't have to be anxious about that any longer. She had found someone she could share her life with. Someone who loves her as much as she loves us."

I smile at Seth, my lips tight, and raise my glass to him.

He nods back at me, smiling pleasantly.

"Welcome to the family, Seth. Welcome also to his sister, Marjorie, and her family." I tip my glass toward the other side of the room, where Marjorie sits.

Marjorie beams, pleased to be the center of attention, just as I knew she would. I've only met Seth's sister a couple of times, but she struck me as shallow and pretentious. I figured she'd like having everyone's eyes on her and on the man sitting next to her, her son, mega-superstar Caleb Lawson. Her husband, Ben, sits meekly behind his wife and child.

"I'll end with a toast to my mother and Seth. I'm so happy that you found each other. Here's to a life filled with endless love. Cheers!"

I raise my glass high above my head and bring it to my lips, taking a sip of white wine. The alcohol washes away any remaining nerves.

Polite applause follows me back to my seat next to Mom.

She leans over and gives me a soft, perfumed kiss on the cheek. "That was wonderful, honey. Thank you."

I nod, knowing it's a compliment that she asked *me*, out of her three children, to give the speech. But really, I'm the obvious choice. Compared to my brothers, Brandon and Teddy, I'm the most stable. The most likely not to be overly stiff and formal like Brandon and not to be too informal and make inappropriate jokes like Teddy.

I glance at the place card in front of my mother's seat. It reads, *Mr. and Mrs. Peterson*. Now we don't even share a last name, my mother and me. It's official. She's moved on, and I'm still here. Stuck. Ever since her engagement, I worry that she'll keep moving on and leave me behind. That I'll lose her, too.

As best man, Caleb is up next to speak. His presence tonight has added an extra sense of excitement to the wedding. The guests have spent as much time gawking at his table as they have looking at the bride and groom.

The crowd hushes, watching him saunter up to the stage. Every eye is trained on him, reverent.

Most celebrities are disappointing when you see them in real life. You realize they aren't as tall as you expected or that they've been photoshopped on the magazine covers.

Not Caleb Lawson.

He's just as handsome in person as he is on the movie screen. He has every attractive feature you can think of: piercing blue eyes, chiseled cheekbones, a full pouty mouth. His hair is the color of sunshine. Like the hazy kind that warms your skin on a tropical beach. Not to mention the muscles. Good grief, those sculpted muscles.

It's all a bit ridiculous, really. That one person should get such a bounty of hotness. Not fair to the rest of us mere mortals.

Microphone in hand, Caleb smiles easily, brilliantly. His teeth are unnaturally white and straight. He's hard to look away from. Something shines out of him beyond his unbelievable good looks. You can see it on the screen when he acts, and it's even more apparent here, when he stands before us. A real-life flesh and blood star.

I'm not the only one who feels it. Women fan themselves in the crowd, and men sit up straighter, smoothing their hair over to the left, just like Caleb's.

I resist the urge to roll my eyes. I've never believed in the idea of celebrity adoration. As far as I'm concerned, movie stars put their pants on one leg at a time, same as the rest of us.

"Good evening, ladies and gentlemen," Caleb begins, voice low and husky.

He pauses, runs his hand through his hair, and swallows. Then his smile widens, and he cracks a joke. "I know it's been an emotional day. The cake is already in tiers."

The crowd laughs uproariously, like he's on a stand-up comedy special.

Which he's not.

"My name is Caleb. Seth is my uncle and godfather. But he's more than that. Seth is my mentor, cheerleader, and conscience. I'm honored that he chose me to stand beside him on this momentous day. The day that he marries his best friend."

The guests all sigh out an "aww," and Caleb glances around the room, smiling sweetly, as if their response is unexpected and charming.

I scoff internally, not understanding why I'm the only one who sees it. That every word out of Caleb's mouth, every quirk of his eyebrow, every gesture of his long-fingered hand is calculated to bring out the most emotional reaction from his audience.

The man is a multi-award-winning actor, for Christ's sakes. Standing in front of a crowd, selling a story, acting. This is what he was raised to do since he was five years old.

Caleb continues. "Preparing this speech has gotten me thinking a lot about love. True love. What does it look like? What does it feel like? Now, I'm obviously no expert, as the tabloids have shown repeatedly." He lets out a small, self-deprecating laugh, and the crowd laughs along with him.

"After some thought, what I came up with is that true love is when someone loves you, even on the days that they don't like you. It's when someone is willing to stand by your side when you are on the top of the world and when the world has crushed you under its heel."

"It's someone who will be there with you for the big things—weddings, birthdays, funerals—and the small things too, taking out the trash, remembering if you prefer tea or coffee. Someone who will take care of you when you are sick or when your feelings are hurt. Someone to kiss away all those casual cruelties that happen in everyday life. Someone who shines a light into your darkness, and you do the same for them. That's what I think about when I say true love."

"Almost a year ago, when Seth first told me that he had found true love, I'm going to be honest with you, I was skeptical. I mean, the man is in his late forties and has never been married. Talk about a red flag!"

More laughter.

"But once I saw them together, Seth and Melinda. Once I saw the way they complement each other's personalities. Well, I don't need to tell you all, because it's apparent from the way they look at each other."

He gestures over at Mom and Seth, his eyes shining, like maybe, just maybe, he might shed a tear.

But he doesn't.

"This, ladies and gentlemen," pausing dramatically, he says. "*This* is true love, and I'm so incredibly grateful that my uncle has found it. May we all be so lucky. Cheers to the happy couple."

The room swells with applause, so loud that it makes the polite clapping I received seem pathetic by comparison.

Caleb grins widely, basking in his moment of glory, before he drains the last of the amber liquor in his glass and struts back to his parents.

The toasts complete, the DJ strikes up some lively music and couples make their way onto the dance floor. Mom and Seth go with them.

I return to Jenny at her table. "It's not fair," I gripe to her. "How am I supposed to compete with Caleb Freaking Lawson? Of course, he's going to give a better toast than I am. He probably had one of his screenwriter friends compose the entire speech for him."

I flop into the seat next to her, looking out the window at the cloudless summer sky. This close to the ocean, the Los Angeles smog gets swept away by the breeze off the water. Palm trees sway outside, teased by that same wind.

Jenny's not listening, too busy staring past me, her eyes wide. "He's coming over here," she says in a breathy whisper, her voice so strangled that I glance over to confirm she's still breathing.

She is. Just barely.

I lift my gaze to the man that has her so excited.

Sure enough, Caleb is walking straight toward us, his eyes fixed on me.

He marches to our table, then stays there, looming over us. I met him briefly before the ceremony, so he knows who I am, but he hasn't spoken with Jenny yet. I make quick introductions.

When he shakes my best friend's hand, she stares up at him unblinking, her mouth hanging open, awestruck. "H—h, h—i, hi. Hello. Hey," Jenny stutters out. I can practically see her brain melting into a puddle of goo. She holds onto his hand for an uncomfortably long time.

My gaze moves to the doors of the ballroom, where two burly men stand with their hands clasped in front of them. Caleb's bodyguards. Seth had warned us they would be here tonight.

I wonder what it's like to be famous, to never truly be alone. I can't imagine it's very pleasant, but it's all that Caleb has ever known. He must be used to it. Who knows? He probably likes it.

The bodyguards watch Jenny's interaction with Caleb closely. As she refuses to let go of his hand, they start to inch toward us. I'm about to warn Jenny when Caleb gently extracts himself from her grip.

"It's nice to meet you," he says smoothly. Then he turns to me. "My mom said I should ask you to dance, seeing how we're family now."

I raise an eyebrow at his request. "Do you usually do what your mother tells you?"

His mouth twitches into a tiny smirk. "Most of the time. I've found it makes my life much easier." He shoves his hands into his pockets, slouching casually, striking a pose like a model on the runway at fashion week. I can't decide if he does that on purpose or if he's truly unaware.

"Well, you can tell her that you asked and I declined," I say primly.

His laugh is startling in its loudness. He squeezes his eyes shut and throws his head back, exposing the long column of his neck, with all of its smooth tan skin. He laughs like I said something hilarious.

I glare at him, annoyed. I wasn't trying to be funny.

The laugh settles down to a chuckle. "That's cute. You obviously haven't spent much time with my mom if you think that's going to satisfy her."

He holds his hand out to me, letting it hang in the air between us, waiting for me to take it.

I don't.

His smirk widens, like he's enjoying the challenge I'm giving him. "I'm going to stand here until you say yes, so you might as well give in."

I hate giving in.

"Look, our moms are united against us." Caleb nods his head toward the other side of the room.

I follow the motion, and, sure enough, my mom stands next to Marjorie. They're staring openly at us. My mom's giving me a pointed glare. I can almost hear her voice in my ear, telling me to "behave."

Fine.

It's her wedding day.

I won't ruin it by making a scene. I take Caleb's hand and rise from my seat.

Leaving an envious Jenny behind, we go to the dance floor. It's a slow song, one that's been on the radio a lot recently.

Caleb tilts his head, listening. "I like this song." He sighs, as if the music pleases him.

He pulls me into him, guiding my arms up around his neck and placing his hands on my waist. I have to rise onto my toes to reach his height. His touch is warm, hot even. Which is weird because a shiver runs through my body at that moment.

We sway together, no fancy dance moves. Caleb is easy to dance with. He leads with expertise, gliding past the other dancers with a firm hand that slides from my waist to the small of my back, drawing me closer. He smells like a mixture of expensive alcohol, scotch or bourbon, and even more expensive cologne, with an undertone of something spicy. Cinnamon, maybe?

After a minute, he bends his head down, so I can hear him over the music. "I heard you're a doctor. That's impressive. Congratulations." He takes a deep inhalation and breathes it back out, tickling my ear.

"Thanks." I readjust my hands around his neck, loosening my fingers and then retightening them for a better grip.

In the past ten years, I've only seen a handful of movies. I've been too busy studying for medical school. But I did see one of his movies. It was a summer blockbuster. I don't fully remember the plot, just that he was a detective and there were a lot of exciting car chases and explosions.

A specific scene stood out to me. It's where he's pulling himself out of the pool. Water pouring off chiseled abs and down his perfect body...

"I heard you're an actor," I say, pretending like I wasn't just picturing his movie... and his body.

He nods, then chuckles darkly when he realizes I won't congratulate him the way he did me.

There's a beat of silence, which he fills by saying, "The ceremony was nice."

"Mmm. Yes. Lovely," I murmur absently, my mind returning to my dad. I wonder what my parents' wedding day was like. What songs were played? It was back in the 1990s, so probably some horrible grunge music. Did they dance together like this, my mother and father?

Caleb must sense my distraction. He pulls apart, just a little, and stares down at me with a quizzical expression, like he's searching for the things I'm not saying.

Up this close, his eyes are aqua blue. Such an unusual color that I search for the rim of contacts, wondering which parts of him are real and which are fake. No contacts that I can see. I squirm slightly, uncomfortable with his scrutiny.

"That was an excellent performance you gave earlier." Without warning, he spins me out away from him. Our arms stretch out taut between us, and then he twitches his wrist and I come back to him, spinning like a top. I crash into his hard chest as he pulls me close.

"Excuse me?" My eyes snap up to his, taking a moment to focus since I'm dizzy from all that twirling.

"The toast you gave. You're a good actress."

I bristle, offended. "That wasn't a performance. Those words were heartfelt and honest." I pull farther away from Caleb, reestablishing the space between us.

"Riiight," he says, making it sound like he means the exact opposite. Like he doesn't believe me. "You can't fool an actor, you know. I can tell you aren't thrilled about your mom marrying my uncle. Is it because you enjoyed having her all to yourself?"

What. The. Heck.

The audacity of this guy.

"First of all, I've never had my mom to myself. I'm the middle child. I always had to share her with my brothers and my dad. And then, after my dad died, I shared her with her work. I don't know what you're talking about, but if I did have any reservations about this wedding, it would have nothing to do with Seth."

I don't understand why I continue. I should stop my rant right there, but the words keep pouring out of me, like they're tired of being bottled up all night. "It's just hard to see her move on. Thirty years ago, my parents said forever in their wedding vows. My dad believed it, but it turned out that his forever was a lot shorter than Mom's, and that makes me sad."

To my horror, there's a prickling in the corners of my eyes, as tears gather there. I look to the ground, hiding them. Caleb's hand is under my chin, lifting it. We're not dancing anymore. Just standing still, staring at each other in the middle of the dance floor.

He's a talented actor, but the sympathy and remorse on his face as he gazes down at me looks awfully sincere. It spears me, the way he's looking at me right now. Like he *sees* me.

"I'm sorry. I'm an ass," he says plainly, like it's a universal truth.

Which, for some reason, makes me laugh, because my emotions are all over the place tonight. Because in all the ways I imagined this wedding going, Caleb Lawson apologizing to me and saying he's an ass wasn't one of them.

It's the first time I've laughed in a long, long while, and it leaves me feeling lighter. Like all my worries are bubbles in a champagne glass, rising to the top to burst and float away into the night.

"Whatever." I roll my eyes at him. "It's fine."

The song ends, as if it thinks we've said enough, and we pull apart.

"Well." There's a hint of awkwardness. "Thanks for the dance." He gives me the tiniest bow.

"Yeah. See you around." I don't know why I say that. He's a busy man. I'll probably never see him again.

We go our separate ways.

I very deliberately don't think about Caleb Lawson again for the rest of the night. And I'm sure he doesn't think about me either…

Available on Amazon and at most major book sellers. FREE to read on Kindle Unlimited.

MEET MELISSA!

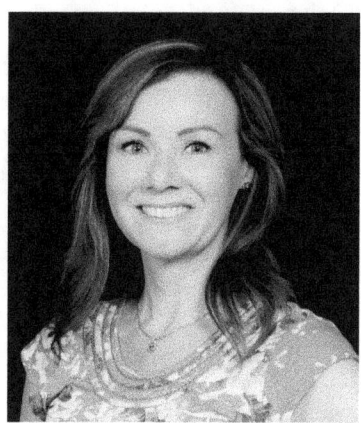

Melissa Dymond is a mom, doctor, and writer.

Born and raised in California, she did her medical school and training in the Midwest. Now she lives in the Southwest surrounded by boys, including her doctor husband, three amazing sons, and an adorable Siberian husky, Buddy.

When she's not working, you can find her drinking an iced white chocolate mocha while voraciously reading, scrolling social media, and planning her family's next Disney vacation.

She would love to connect with you on her website, www.melissadymondauthor.com, where you can sign up for her newsletter, get free chapters and writing updates, see character art, get the best deals on bookish merchandise, and share book related-memes.

Also, she would love to chat with you on social media, where she spends WAY too much time. Join her at:

Instagram: https://www.instagram.com/melissadymondauthor
Facebook: https://www.facebook.com/melissadymondauthor
Tiktok: https://www.tiktok.com/@melissadymond6

GLOSSARY

PATH TO BECOMING A DOCTOR

Medical student: After completing four years of college, these students go on to medical school, which lasts four years. The first two years are spent in the classroom. During the last two years, students do clinical rotations in hospitals and clinics.

Typically, they spend a month at a time doing various specialties of medicine. For example, a student may work a month in the surgery department, a month doing internal medicine, a month in a pediatrics clinic, and so on.

These clinical rotations serve two purposes: 1) for the students to gain a broad understanding of how different types of doctors practice, and 2) so students can test out different types of medicine in order to choose which they like best. They will then apply for a residency in that preferred specialty.

Note: Medical students wear short white lab coats to distinguish them from doctors who have graduated from medical school. Once they graduate, they are allowed to wear long white lab coats.

Intern: The first year of training after graduating from medical school is called internship. Since the individuals have graduated from medical school, they are doctors. They have certain privileges not allowed to medical students, such as prescribing medications and performing procedures. However, they are still in training and are supervised by attending physicians. Most internships have the same rotating structure as the last two years of medical school, with interns spending a month at a time in different departments and clinics.

Resident: After completing their internship year, doctors go on to their residency. This is where they will specialize and train to become a specific type of doctor. For example, a doctor can do a family practice residency and then work as a primary care physician, or a doctor may do an emergency medicine residency and work in the Emergency Room. Residency can last anywhere from three to six years (including the internship year). Residents are labeled as a first-year resident, second-year resident, and so on.

Fellow: After graduating from residency, some doctors do a fellowship where they sub-specialize in their specific field of medicine. Fellowships can last from one to three years. For example, to become a cardiologist, a doctor completes a three-year internal medicine residency followed by a three-year cardiology fellowship.

Attending physician: Often just called attendings, these are doctors who have completed all of their medical training and work autonomously. If they wish, attending physicians can be involved in training and teaching younger generations of doctors (medical students, interns, residents, or fellows).

ACKNOWLEDGMENTS

Hello, Dear Reader,

Before I get to the acknowledgments, I have to tell you that I AGONIZED over what Tiffany should do with the diamonds. I spent weeks discussing the pros and cons of each option with my husband, friends, even the barista at my coffee shop! My beta readers' strong opinions on the topic didn't help either. Half of them argued that Tiffany should give the diamonds to Stewart, while the other half advocated for Tiffany to destroy them.

In the end, I tried to reach a compromise that I felt reflected Tiffany's own conflicted feelings, where she got rid of the diamonds but still brought some as a gift to Stewart to assuage her guilty conscience. I hope you found that solution satisfying. If you didn't, you can always email me (hello@melissadymondauthor.com) with your preferred ending, and I can email you ALL three endings that I wrote when I was trying to figure it out. Lol!

The other thing I want to say is that I love Las Vegas! In this novel I make it sound shady and grim, but that is a plot device, not a statement about real-life Las Vegas. I wanted there to be an ominous, unsafe feeling when you were in the past chapters and to contrast that with the hard-won stability that Tiffany had forged for herself in the present-day chapters. I've been going to Las Vegas since I was young and even had the privilege of living there for two months working in local hospitals when I was a medical student. If you are a fan of Las Vegas, please don't feel offended by my less-than-favorable portrayal of it in this book.

Okay, all that's out of the way. Now, on to the acknowledgments. I can't believe I'm writing the acknowledgments for my second book! I had SO much fun with my first novel, *Holiday Star,* thanks to readers like you. Now, we get to do it all over again with this book.

The first person I want to thank is YOU, dear reader. You have literally made my dreams come true by picking up this book and reading it. Please know how much I appreciate you. Thanks also to those of you who choose to leave a review, post on social media, send me an email or a DM, and recommend my books to your friends and family. Those extra steps are above and beyond. I can't express how much they mean to me. You are an amazing, brilliant, wonderful human being, and I am eternally grateful to you.

I'm fortunate that I've met some talented people who helped make this book shine. Thank you to my editor, Caroline Acebo, for your insightful critique and suggestions. Thank you to my mother, who is also my copyeditor. I couldn't do this without you. Thank you for being patient while formatting this book, Steve Kuhn. Thank you to my cover and art designers at Qamber Design, who let me email them crazy endless art requests. Thank you for my gorgeous website, Katharine Bolin. Seriously, this website is so pretty! www.melissadymondauthor.com

Thank you to all the wonderful and supportive friends I have had through the years: Michelle Center, Judy Fann, Karen Fann, Tricia Verhoeven, Charity Yarnal, Pam Noll, Janelle McGough, Nicole Danner, Jen Julian, Jenn Hamilton, Marcie Lane, Nicole Rempfer, Julie Sallquist, Liz Martin, Jill Rother, Jackie Hernandez, Camila Parris, Maren Umlauf, Collin Zaffery, Stephanie Horton, Parris Maxwell, Darren Todd, Dorene McLaughlin, Jenna Price, Laura Weiss Ross, and so many more.

Thank you to Tina Marshall who is a bright light in the book community. I appreciate your continued support and how generous you are with your knowledge.

Thanks to my family. My talented mother, who inspired my love of writing. My dad, who sat next to me watching Saturday morning cartoons and thus inspired a love of stories filled with laughter and drama. Love to my beautiful sister-in-law Amelia and her awesome husband Steven.

Most of all, love to my three sons, who are the absolute center of my universe. Being your mom has brought me more joy than I ever thought was possible. Love also to my husband, Andrew. Once upon a time I had to train a cocky and annoyingly handsome (the nurses all called him Dr. McDreamy—picture me rolling my eyes right now) radiology resident. This story is our love story. The best story of all.

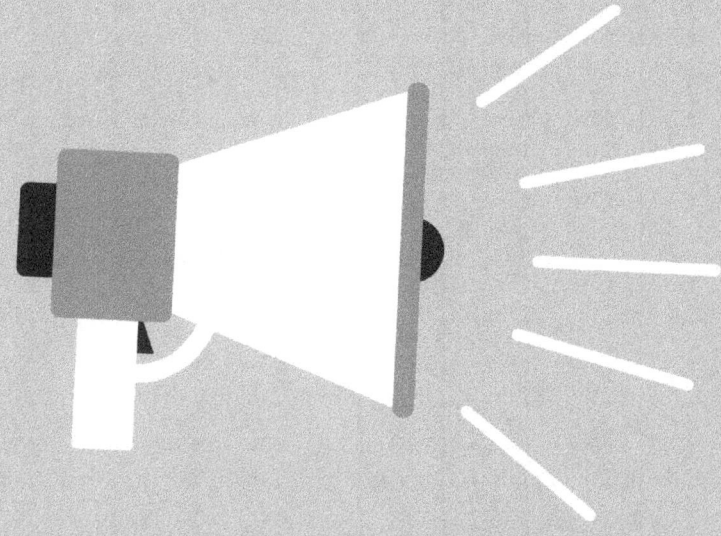

Check out my website and join my newsletter for exciting updates about writing, book releases, great book deals, freebies, and more.

WWW.MELISSADYMONDAUTHOR.COM

www.ingramcontent.com/pod-product-compliance
Lightning Source LLC
LaVergne TN
LVHW010307070526
838199LV00065B/5468